HEPATITIS B:
A SEXUALLY TRANSMITTED DISEASE
IN HETEROSEXUALS

HEPATITIS B: A SEXUALLY TRANSMITTED DISEASE IN HETEROSEXUALS

Proceedings of a Symposium held in Barcelona, 6–7 May 1990

Editors:

P. PIOT and **F.E. ANDRE**

1990

EXCERPTA MEDICA, AMSTERDAM – NEW YORK – OXFORD

International Congress Series No. 919
ISBN 0 444 81356 x

This book is printed on acid-free paper.

Published by:
Elsevier Science Publishers B.V.
(Biomedical Division)
P.O. Box 211
1000 AE Amsterdam
The Netherlands

Sole distributors for the USA and Canada:
Elsevier Science Publishing Company Inc.
655 Avenue of the Americas
New York, NY 10010
USA

Library of Congress Cataloging–in–Publication Data

Hepatitis B : a sexually transmitted disease in heterosexuals : proceedings of a symposium held in Barcelona, 6-7 May 1990 / editors, P. Piot and F.E. André.
p. cm. -- (International congress series ; no. 919)
Includes index.
ISBN 0-444-81356-X (alk. paper)
1. Hepatitis B--Transmission--Congresses. 2. Hepatitis B--Epidemiology--Congresses. I. André, F. E. II. Piot, Peter, 1949- . III. Series.
[DNLM: 1. Hepatitis B--prevention & control--congresses. 2. Hepatitis B--transmission--congresses. 3. Sexually Transmitted Diseases--congresses. W3 EX89 no. 919 / WC 536 H5335 1990]
RC848.H44H483 1990
616.3'623--dc20
DNLM/DLC
for Library of Congress 90-14089
CIP

This volume has been prepared using the newly developed method of electronic text processing, generally known as Desk Top Publishing. In order to ensure rapid publication, while at the same time maintaining the highest degree of scientific accuracy and consistency of style, the manuscripts have only been subjected to basic linguistic editing.

Printed in The Netherlands

CONTENTS

STDs AND HEPATITIS B

© 1990 Elsevier Science Publishers B.V. (Biomedical Division)
Hepatitis B: A sexually transmitted disease in heterosexuals.
P. Piot and F.E. Andre, editors

Sex-related aspects of hepatitis B infection and its consequences

BARUCH S. BLUMBERG

Balliol College, Oxford 0X1 3BJ, England, UK, and Fox Chase Cancer Center, Philadelphia, USA

Introduction

Soon after the discovery of the hepatitis B virus (HBV), there were occasional observations within families from which it was inferred that heterosexual transmission of HBV was a common event. If one member of a connubial pair was a carrier of HBV, his or her partner had a much higher probability of having anti-HBs than an individual randomly chosen from the population. It was also found that the probability that the mate of a HBV carrier would become a carrier was not much greater than expectation. This was consistent with the explanation that, whereas there is a high risk of infection in a sexual partner of a carrier, there is an additional requirement (possibly genetic) to increase the probability that the partner would develop the carrier state (1). With increasing experience it became more apparent that sexual activity may be one of the most common forms of HBV transmission, particularly in regions of moderate or low endemicity of HBV. Appropriate public health and health education steps are now being taken to decrease the probability of transmission through this route.

Sexual transmission of hepatitis B and vaccination

It is likely that, overall, HBV is transmitted sexually more commonly than HIV. In the case of HBV a safe and effective vaccine is available; unfortunately this is not so for HIV. An obvious solution to sexual transmission of HBV would be universal vaccination which included adolescents and adults. This is unlikely to occur before infant vaccination programs are more advanced, although in some countries these programs will develop sooner. Individuals can undertake vaccination independent of public health programs, and in many cases will probably do so.

Sex-related aspects of hepatitis B infection

Consequences of HBV infection such as acute hepatitis, fulminant hepatitis, chronic persistent or active hepatitis, liver cirrhosis and hepatocellular carcinoma have been well studied and are generally known. Some aspects of the consequences of HBV infection have not, however, been the subject of intensive research, but nevertheless are of considerable biological and possibly Public Health importance. They are related to sex but not only in the literal sense.

Nearly everything about hepatitis B infection and host responses to it are sex related. When infected, males are much more likely to become carriers and females to develop anti-HBs (2). Males are likely to remain carriers longer than females. In most populations the ratio of male to female carriers is about two or greater (see for example ref. 3). Following treatment with interferon, females are more likely to respond than males. It has been inferred that male carriers are more likely to develop primary hepatocellular carcinoma (PHC) than female carriers and the ratio of males to females among patients with primary carcinoma can be 5 or higher in most populations.

For obvious reasons the female carrier parent is more likely to transmit HBV to a child than the male carrier parent (4). The mother may transmit HBV *in utero* or at the time of birth. After delivery mothers in most societies have more social interaction with their children than do fathers, and this increases the probability of maternal transmission. We have compared the transmission of HBV within families in village communities in Senegal. Transmission was most likely to occur from mothers to children, next from sibs to sibs, and transmission from fathers to children was not greatly different from random transmission from outside the family (5). There was a different pattern in a traditionally male homosexual community in the Pacific where there were correlations indicating that male to male transmission was a common transmission mode (6).

HBV infection and sex ratio

One of the most curious sex differences for HBV was uncovered during a family study conducted in a community in Macedonia in Northern Greece in 1973 (7). We had been interested in family studies since our earliest investigations of the genetics of the carrier state (8). Sera were collected from most of the inhabitants of the town and tested for HBsAg and anti-HBs. The results were analyzed by family groupings according to the response of parents following exposure to HBV. We found that, if one of the parents was a carrier (families with both parent carriers were uncommon) then the sex ratio (defined as the number of male offspring divided by the number of female offspring times 100) was higher than in families in which the parents were not carriers. In a subsequent analysis we found the sex ratio was highest in HBsAg(+) carriers, lowest in families in which the parents (in particular the mother) was anti-HBs and intermediate in families in which the parents were uninfected (9). In this population both the carrier and anti-HBs families had about the same number of boys, but had fewer girls. The carrier families therefore have fewer children and fewer girls than the anti-HBs; hence, there is an effect both on sex ratio and family size.

We have postulated several biological and behavioral explanations for these findings. The observations could be explained by the relatively decreased viability of a female compared to a male conceptus infected with or exposed to HBV. There could also be a behavioral component. In societies where male children are valued more than females, there is often a desire to have a certain number of male offspring. In the carrier families, there is a high probability of producing boys; from our data, about 2 appears to be the favoured number. Hence the carrier parents stop producing children after the desired number is achieved. However, the anti-HBs families are more likely to have girls, and they continue to have children until they have the desired number of boys, ending up with a larger family with more girls than the carrier parents.

Because of the curious nature of these findings we have attempted to validate them in other populations, including Papua New Guinea (10), The Philippines (11) and Greenland (12). The sex-ratio difference observed in Greece was confirmed in the other populations. There has been some confirmation from other laboratories but the problem has, for the most part, remained unstudied.

Iron, ferritin, HBV infection and sex

We have completed a large number of studies on serum iron, ferritin and transferrin in relation to HBV infection and its outcome. These have been extended to population studies of mortality in general, and morbidity and mortality from cancer, but these are not relevant to the present paper and will not be discussed further (13). Carriers of HBV have higher levels of iron than individuals who are uninfected (14-16). In a study in Senegal the difference was found to be most striking in females. In the tropical regions where HBV is common, iron is often deficient in the diet and hemoglobin levels are, on average, lower than in temperate regions. One could conjecture that the HBV carrier state may be relatively advantageous in that given the same level of dietary iron intake, the carriers would retain more iron. This would be particularly valuable in females who, between menstruation and menopause, loose blood regularly and require more iron than men. In previous times, when life expectancy was lower than at present, the HBV carrier state was probably less of a disadvantage. Carriers would usually die from other causes before the effects of chronic HBV infection could shorten life as a consequence of chronic liver disease and primary hepatocellular carcinoma.

We have also investigated the relation between serum ferritin levels and the probability of becoming a hepatitis B carrier following exposure to HBV (17). Previously, several factors have been shown to increase the probability of becoming a carrier. These include: (1) age, the young are more likely to become carriers than older people, (2) sex, males are more likely to become carriers than females, and (3) some sort of genetic predisposition. There is now a growing body of data that HLA types and immune states of the host may be related to the probability of carrier state development.

Ferritin levels may be another factor. The study of ferritin was conducted in a renal dialysis unit in Philadelphia beginning in the early 1970's. At that time, blood screening for HBV was not done and HBV infection was a frequent consequence of renal dialysis and the blood transfusion associated with it. We had stored serum samples from renal dialysis patients before, at about the time of, and after infection with HBV. We tested the hypotheses that individuals who had higher ferritin levels before infection were more likely to become carriers than those with lower ferritin levels and that those with the lower ferritin levels were more likely to develop anti-HBs. The data supported the hypothesis and we concluded that in this population, increased ferritin levels (which might be an indicator of total body iron stores) increased the probability that an infected individual would develop the carrier state.

In later studies (18) we found that, in patients with chronic hepatitis B infection, those who went on to develop PHC were more likely to have had elevated ferritin and decreased transferrin levels than the patients who did not develop PHC within the observation period. A variety of studies in mice have confirmed these original impressions and have been extended to the relation of increased ferritin and decreased albumin levels to the more rapid development of cancers in general.

Transmission of HBV by bedbugs and other insects

There is another body of information which has an unusual relation to sexual activity. There has been a considerable interest in the possibility of insect transmission of HBV. Several studies on mosquitoes have shown that there is a high field infection rate (of the order of 1:200) and that detectable virus may remain in the mosquitoes for several weeks after a blood meal (19–22).

In Senegal we collected bed bugs (*Cimex hemipterus*) from beds whose main occupants were carriers of HBV. More than sixty percent of the insects had detectable HBsAg (23, 24). After a single feed of HBsAg(+) blood, HBsAg could be detected in the body of the insect for up to 6 weeks and in the faeces for 2 weeks after the cessation of a blood meal. The infected faeces accumulates as dust in the bed and, theoretically could enter the blood stream of another occupant through ulcerous or other lesions on the skin. Hence, virus could be transmitted to another occupant of the bed, i.e. a child or sexual partner. In the latter case, it represents an unusual form of 'venereal' transmission. There was no evidence that replication occurred either in the bed bugs or mosquitos.

An international controlled study is now in progress in the Gambia to determine if systematic insect control can decrease HBV infection. When complete this could provide important information of potential public health importance. A final item concerning HBV and sex. In the experiment with bed bugs, it was found that the female imbibes more blood than does the male (25).

Conclusion

Sexual transmission is undoubtedly an important mechanism for the perpetuation of HBV in human populations. An understanding of the complex relation of HBV to human sex differences will reveal a great deal of important information of biological value, but also help in developing appropriate mechanisms of control.

References

1. Blumberg BS, Melartin L, Guinto RA, and Werner B, (1966) Am J Human Genet, 18: 594.
2. London WT and Drew JS (1977) Proc Natl Acad Sci (U.S.A.) 74: 2561.
3. Blumberg BS, Sutnick AI, London WT and Melartin L (1972) Arch Intern Med 130: 227.
4. Larouzé B, London WT, Saimot G, Werner BB, Lustbader ED, Payet M and Blumberg BS (1976) Lancet 2: 534.
5. Marinier E, Barrois V, Larouzé B, London WT, Cofer A, Diakhate L and Blumberg BS (1984) In: Immunita ed Infezione Nelle Malattie del Fegato e del Tratto Gastroenterico del Bambino, Ed. A. Vierucci. Masson Italia Editori S.p.A., Milano, pp. 379.
6. Langendorfer A, Davenport E, London WT, Blumberg BS and Mazzur S (1984) Am J Phys Anthropol 64: 243.
7. Hesser JE, Economidou J and Blumberg BS (1975) Human Biol. 47: 415.
8. Blumberg BS, Melartin L, Guinto RA, and Werner B (1966) Am J Human Genet, 18: 594.
9. Drew JS, London WT, Lustbader ED, Hesser JE and Blumberg BS (1978) Science 201: 687.
10. Drew J, London WT, Blumberg BS and Serjeantson S (1982) Human Biology 54: 123.

11. London WT, Stevens RG, Shofer FS. Drew JS, Brunhofer JE and Blumberg BS. (1982) In: Viral Hepatitis, 1981 International Symposium. Eds W Szmuness, H. J. Alter and J. E. Maynard Franklin Institute Press, Philadelphia, p. 195.
12. Drew JS, Blumberg BS and Robert-Lamblin, J (1986) Human Biology 58: 115.
13. Blumberg BS (1986) In: Viruses, Immunity and Immunodeficiency. Ed A. Szentivanyi and H. Friedman. Plenum Publishing Corp, New York, p. 81.
14. Sutnick AI, Blumberg BS and Lustbader ED (1974) Ann. Internal Med. 81: 855.
15. Felton C, Lustbader BD, Merten C and Blumberg, BS (1979) Proc. Natl. Acad. Sci. USA 76: 2438.
16. Blumberg BS, Lustbader ED and Whitford, PL (1981) Proc Natl Acad Sci USA 78: 3222.
17. Lustbader ED, Hann HL and Blumberg, BS (1983) Science 220: 423.
18. Hann HL, Kim CY, London WT and Blumberg BS (1989) Int J. Cancer 43: 376.
19. Wills W, Saimot G, Brochard C, Blumberg BS, London WT, Dechene R and Millman I (1976) Am J Trop Med Hyg 25: 186.
20. Blumberg BS, Wills W, Millman I and London WT (1973) Res Commun Chem Path Pharm 6: 719.
21. Metselaar D, Blumberg BS, Millman I, Parker AM and Bagshawe AF (1973) Lancet 2: 758.
22. Wills W, Larouze B, London WT, Millman I, Werner BG, Ogston W, Pourtaghva M, Diallo S and Blumberg BS (1977) Lancet 2: 217.
23. Ogston CW, Wittenstein FS, London WT and Millman I (1979) J Infect Dis 140: 411.
24. Ogston CW and London WT (1980) Trans Roy Soc Trop Med Hyg 74: 823.
25. Yanovski AD and Ogston CW (1982) J Med Entomol 19: 45.

Transmission of the hepatitis B virus in areas of low endemicity

MARK A. KANE

Microbiology and Immunology Support Services, Division of Communicable Diseases, World Health Organization, 1211 Geneva 27, Switzerland

INTRODUCTION

Epidemiological studies have permitted the definition of regions of endemicity of hepatitis B infection (1). Most of Africa, Asia and the Amazon Basin can be considered as zones of high endemicity - most adults have serological evidence of previous hepatitis B infection and more than 10% of the population in these areas are chronic carriers of the virus. In regions of low endemicity (North America, Western Europe and Australia, for example), most people do not come into contact with the virus and fewer than 2% of the population are chronic carriers. This does not mean that hepatitis B is not an important cause of morbidity in low endemicity areas. In the United States, hepatitis B is the fourth most commonly reported notifiable viral disease (2). In addition, only a small proportion of the true number of infections are reported, as many cases of hepatitis B are asymptomatic. The Centers for Disease Control (CDC) estimated that in 1987 there were approximately 300,000 cases of infection and half of these were asymptomatic. There were about 18 to 30,000 persons who became chronic carriers; 4000 deaths were caused by hepatitis B-related cirrhosis and 800 by hepatitis B related primary liver cancer (3). Significant subpopulations of countries such as the US have endemic levels of hepatitis B infection. Recent studies have shown that a far greater proportion of blacks in the US had been infected with the hepatitis B virus as compared to whites (4). Indeed, in the 55-60 year age group, approximately 40% of blacks had serological evidence of infection, although the overall percentage of Americans infected is only 5%.

These differences in epidemiology led to the development of different strategies for the control of hepatitis B once a vaccine against this disease became available. The strategies were based on the primary modes of transmission in each area of endemicity. In areas of intermediate to high endemicity where transmission is primarily perinatal or child-to-child, it was decided that all infants should receive hepatitis B vaccine as pre-exposure prophylaxis. In the countries where it could be afforded, maternal screening could be carried out, with the administration of hepatitis B immuneglobulin (HBIg) for the infants of HBsAg-positive mothers. In areas of low endemicity, it was thought that the proper strategy for the control of hepatitis B was to give vaccine to individuals in groups at high risk for the disease. Recent evidence suggests that this strategy will not lead to the control of this infection, and universal infant immunization will be required everywhere.

Modes of viral transmission in countries of low endemicity and definition of groups at risk

Since 1973, transfusion with infected blood as a cause of infection has been drastically reduced in North America and Western Europe, due to efficient screening techniques. Many developing countries have yet to establish routine, sensitive screening for HBsAg in blood.

The use of contaminated needles can also spread hepatitis B. In Europe and the US, this mode of transmission is essentially observed in intravenous drug abusers. In many other parts of the world, however, rigorous sterilization of needles, syringes and medical equipment is not performed. The reuse of unsterilized equipment may be an important factor in the propagation of both hepatitis B and HIV to children in the developing world. Two recent outbreaks of hepatitis B occurring in orphanages in the Soviet Union and Rumania, have shown that proper sterilization does not always take place in these areas.

Perinatal transmission is very important for a number of reasons. In most instances, transmission of the virus occurs at the time of birth rather than *in utero* (5), which permits prophylaxis of infected newborns using hepatitis B vaccine with or without HBIg. The outcome of infection in newborns is very different from adults, where most cases of hepatitis B infection resolve and only between 6 - 10% of all infections lead to chronic carriage. The infected newborn has a much greater chance of becoming a chronic carrier than the adult; about 75 - 90% of infected newborns will be shown to be carriers between the ages of 1 to 2 years (6,7). Moreover, in young children, virtually all hepatitis B infections are subclinical; the child does not become ill or jaundiced and infections are not noticed by the parents or physicians. In studies carried out in Taiwan, it has been estimated that overall 25% of individuals who become chronic hepatitis B virus carriers in childhood will die of the sequelae of infection such as chronic cirrhosis or hepatoma (8). This figure may be as high as 40% for men.

In the developing countries, the most important mode of transmission is from child to child, probably via skin lesions. Damaged skin, due to impetigo, insect bites or cuts and scratches, means that the virus can be present on the skin of a carrier child and be passed through contact during play to the skin of susceptible children. In developed countries, this type of transmission is less common. However, in the development of national recommendations for the prevention of disease, doctors from the US or Europe residing in Africa, Asia or the Pacific Basin, often look to their own countries for guidance. It is therefore important that this mode of transmission not be overlooked.

In the US, health care workers account for 12,000 cases of hepatitis B infection per year, making this disease the major infectious occupational health hazard in these individuals. The US Occupational Safety and Health Administration (OSHA) takes hepatitis B very seriously and has developed stringent rules to ensure the vaccination of most health care workers in the US. Transmission of the hepatitis B virus usually occurs from patients to health care personnel (9,10), but there have been cases of transmission from health care personnel to patients. Many of these outbreaks were due to oral surgery and one involved over 50 patients (11-13). Outbreaks such as these can destroy the career of the doctor or dentist, and in large part, can be prevented by vaccination.

The sexual transmission of the hepatitis B virus may be responsible for nearly one-third of all cases of hepatitis B per year reported in the US (14). This mode of transmission will be amply discussed in other papers (this volume).

Immigrants from areas of high endemicity to regions of low prevalence

Approximately 1 million refugees from Asia have migrated to the US during the past several years. Do the ways that the hepatitis B virus is transmitted change when a 'high incidence' population moves to a 'low incidence' area? A recent study of US-born children of Indochinese refugees was designed to explore this question (15). Approximately 90% of the children of HBeAg+ carrier mothers had been infected with the hepatitis B virus and about 60% had become chronic carriers, showing that these children were not being adequately protected against infection, even though they were born in the US. High rates of chronic carriage were also found in what were considered as infants at low risk of infection. A child of a non-carrier mother who had a sibling who was a carrier had approximately a 25% chance of being infected with hepatitis B; evidence of infection was found in 5% of children with no apparent household exposure.

Several studies have shown that the risk to household contacts of adopted carrier children from endemic areas is also high (16, 17). These children should be screened, and if shown to be hepatitis B virus carriers, their adoptive families should receive vaccine.

Vaccination strategies for groups at 'high risk'

In the US, the policy of vaccinating groups of individuals perceived to be at risk for hepatitis B infection has not resulted in a decrease in the incidence of disease. Indeed, since the introduction of vaccine in the US in 1982, the incidence of hepatitis B actually increased but has more recently leveled off (1). Most individuals at high risk of infection are in contact with the hepatitis B virus before they can be vaccinated; for example, 60 - 90% of all intravenous drug abusers have been infected by the time they seek medical help (18). In addition, these individuals are unlikely to be interested in preventative medicine.

The importance of perinatal infection as a cause of the chronic carrier state led to the development of programs for the prophylaxis of neonates of HBsAg-positive carrier mothers. It had been shown that the administration of HBIg and hepatitis B vaccine to these neonates could reduce the incidence of chronic carriage to less than 15% (19, 20). In 1984, health care workers who attended to pregnant women were asked, on the basis of race and several other factors which would make them at high risk of carriage, to evaluate whether a given woman was a potential carrier. These women were then screened, and if they were carriers, their infants administered HBIg and hepatitis B vaccine. This strategy failed for a number of reasons. First, many health care workers did not know enough about the epidemiology of hepatitis B to know which women they saw required screening. In addition, subsequent studies showed that only 35–50% of the carrier women in US inner cities actually belong to a 'high-risk group'. The strategy consisting of the selective screening of women thought to be in high risk groups and the vaccination of infants of carrier mothers is therefore not effective in halting the transmission of the hepatitis B virus. The Immunization Practice Advisory Committee (ACIP) recommended that all women be tested for HBsAg at an early prenatal visit (21), and has now recommended vaccination for all infants of women from highly endemic areas (3).

Since 1982, about 85% of the hepatitis B vaccine administered in the United States and Europe has been given to health care workers, yet this group represents less than 5% of all cases of hepatitis B. Indeed, data from the CDC has demonstrated that a large proportion of all cases of hepatitis B are of unknown origin (22). This 'group' is therefore difficult to reach in vaccination campaigns aimed at groups at high risk.

Conclusions

Certainly, good medical care implies giving vaccine to health care workers and others at high risk of infection but this will not be enough to control the spread of the virus in a given country.

Ultimately, vaccine will have to be administered to infants or, in some countries, adolescents, to ensure good vaccine coverage. Young children are routinely brought by their parents for vaccination; the infrastructure for the delivery of vaccines to infants is usually good. The vaccination of adolescents may be added to infant immunization in countries where more rapid control of hepatitis B infection can be afforded. The control of hepatitis B in countries of low endemicity will only follow mass vaccination of infants and adolescents rather than selective vaccination of individuals considered at risk.

References

1. Centers for Disease Control (1989) Hepatitis Surveillance, report 52.
2. US Department of Health and Human Services (1989) MMWR 37(54): 1.
3. Immunization Practices Advisory Committee (1990) MMWR 39(S-2): 1.
4. McQuillan GM, Townsend TR, Fields HA, Carroll M, Leahy M, Polk F (1989) Am J Med 87(3A): 5S.
5. Stevens CE, Beasley RP, Tsui J, Lee WC (1987) N Engl J Med 292: 771.
6. Beasley RP, Hwang L-Y, Lee GC-Y et al (1983) Lancet ii: 1099.
7. Chung WK, Yoo JY,Sun HS et al (1985) J Infect Dis 151: 280.
8. Beasley RP, Hwang L-Y, Lin CC, Chien CS (1981) Lancet ii: 1129.
9. Christenson B (1985) Am J Epidemiol 122: 411.
10. Osterholm MT, Garayalde SM (1985) JAMA 254: 3207.
11. Rimland D, Parkin W, Miller GB, Schrack WD (1977) N Engl J Med 296: 953.
12. Shaw FE, Barrett CL, Hamm R et al (1986) JAMA 255: 3260.
13. Welch J, Webster M, Tilzey AJ, Noah ND, Banatvala JE (1989) Lancet i: 205.
14. Anonymous (1988) MMWR 37(28): 429.
15. Franks AL, Berg CJ, Kane MA et al (1989) N Engl J Med 321: 1301.
16. Friede A, Harris JR, Kobayashi JM, Shaw FE, Shoemaker-Nawas PC, Kane MA (1988) Am J Public Health 78: 26.
17. Hershow RC, Hadler SC, Kane MA (1987) Pediatr Infect Dis J 6: 431.
18. Kane MA, Alter MJ, Hadler SC, Margolis HS (1989) Am J Med 87(3A): 11S.
19. Lo K-J, Tsai Y-T, Lee S-D et al (1985) J Infect Dis 152: 817.
20. Stevens CE, Toy PT, Tong MJ et al (1985) JAMA 253: 1740.

21. Immunization Practices Advisory Committee (1988) MMWR 37(22): 341.
22. Alter MJ, Hadler SC, Margolis HS et al (1990) JAMA 263: 1218.

HETEROSEXUAL TRANSMISSION OF HEPATITIS B

© 1990 Elsevier Science Publishers B.V. (Biomedical Division)
Hepatitis B: A sexually transmitted disease in heterosexuals.
P. Piot and F.E. Andre , editors

Heterosexual activity: A leading risk factor in the transmission of hepatitis B

MIRIAM J. ALTER

Hepatitis Branch, Centers for Disease Control, Building 6, Room 154 (A-33), Atlanta, GA 30333, USA

Introduction

Worldwide, chronic hepatitis B virus (HBV) infection is a major cause of chronic hepatitis, cirrhosis, and primary hepatocellular carcinoma (1). In those countries where HBV is highly endemic, it is primarily an infection of infants and children (1). In countries with low rates of infection, transmission during infancy and childhood is uncommon, and sexual transmission is important in the spread of this disease. In the United States, it is estimated that 300,000 HBV infections occur annually (2). These primarily occur in young adults with certain behavioral, occupational or life-style associated risk factors. Sexual activity, both homosexual and heterosexual, is the most commonly reported risk factor for HBV infection. Since 1985, however, the number of cases of hepatitis B in homosexual men has declined by 62%; in contrast, the number of cases of hepatitis B due to heterosexual activity has increased by 38% (3). Heterosexual activity now accounts for at least 25% of cases and has replaced homosexual activity in importance as a risk factor for hepatitis B.

Sexual transmission from acute hepatitis B cases or chronic carriers

Transmission of HBV from persons with acute or chronic hepatitis B to their sexual partners is an important source of infection. Several studies have reported the transmission of HBV from patients with acute hepatitis B to their sexual partners. The risk of infection was shown to range from 20% to 42% when susceptible heterosexual partners of persons with acute hepatitis B were followed for 3 to 12 months after identification of the index case (4-6).

There is also a high risk of HBV infection among the sexual contacts of persons chronically infected with HBV. Studies have shown that the prevalence of serologic markers indicating past or present HBV infection is 2 to 10 times higher among the household (including sexual) contacts of HBV carriers than among such contacts of non-carriers (7-11). In two of these studies, spouses or other sexual partners of HBV carriers had a higher prevalence of HBV infection than did other members of the household (8, 9).

Heterosexual activity has also been associated with outbreaks of acute hepatitis B. In a small outbreak of HBV infections in a nursing home in 1973, the only exposure identified for two of the three cases was sexual contact with an HBV carrier (12). Among a cluster of 31 cases of hepatitis B in south Wales (13), the index case, a male parenteral drug user, transmitted HBV to three needle sharing contacts. One of these contacts (a woman) subsequently transmitted HBV to four non-drug using sexual partners as well as to an additional 17 needle sharing contacts. Six of these contacts transmitted HBV to their sexual partners.

In non-outbreak situations, the source for patients with acute hepatitis B may often be sexual exposure to clinically ill or a symptomatic hepatitis B surface antigen (HBsAg)-positive contacts. Heathcote et al. (14) investigated 67 patients with acute hepatitis B admitted to London hospitals to determine the source for their infection. Only 16 admitted to parenteral exposures; of the remaining 51, 13 had sexual exposure to contacts who were either jaundiced or HBsAg-positive, and 12 had household (non-sexual) exposure to a contact with a history of jaundice or who was HBsAg-positive. Papaevangelou et al. (15) investigated the possible source of infection in 260 patients hospitalized for acute hepatitis B in Greece. For 132 patients, no parenteral source of infection could be identified; 30 of these were found to have a sexual partner who was HBsAg-positive (and asymptomatic) or who had a history of acute hepatitis B in the 2 to 6 months preceeding onset of illness in their partners. In the United States, surveillance for cases of acute hepatitis B in four counties found that among patients with no known parenteral exposures, approximately 35% acquired disease from sexual partners who had had a recent episode of acute hepatitis B or who were HBsAg-positive but asymptomatic and were detected through serologic testing of contacts (3).

Risk factors for transmission of HBV through heterosexual activity

The same factors associated with an increased risk of HBV infection in homosexual men, i.e., multiple partners, duration of sexual activity, and history of other sexually transmitted diseases, have been found to be associated with an increased risk of HBV infection in heterosexual men and women. Two prevalence studies have found an association between HBV infection and number of recent sexual partners (Table I). One of these (16) found that heterosexual women attending a sexually transmitted disease (STD) clinic who had a history of 3 or more partners in the preceding 6 month period were more likely to have evidence of HBV infection (18%) than women with less than 3 partners (1%). No such association was found for heterosexual men, and other risk factors associated with HBV infection were not accounted for. For both white men and women attending an STD clinic in the United States with no history of other risk factors for hepatitis B, increasing numbers of recent (in the preceding 4 months) partners were associated with a 4-fold risk of HBV infection (17). Among a group of white students attending a large coeducational university and accessed during a school-wide blood donor drive in this same study, the overall prevalence of HBV infection was only 2%; however, students with 3 or more partners in the preceding 4 months had a prevalence of 14%, 11-fold higher than students with fewer than 3 partners. Among persons with acute hepatitis B, two case-control studies have demonstrated that having recent multiple heterosexual partners is significantly associated with acquiring acute disease in persons with no other commonly recognized exposures (18, CDC, unpublished data).

Number of lifetime sexual partners has also been associated with HBV infection (Table II). Studies conducted in heterosexual men and women attending STD clinics have found a direct relationship between increasing number of lifetime partners and increasing risk of HBV infection reaching 20% to 30% in those with the greatest number of partners (17,19). Number of lifetime partners has also been associated with an increased risk of HBV infection among university students who had no other risk factors for hepatitis B (17). In this group, the prevalence of HBV infection was 7% in students with 10 or more lifetime partners compared with 2% in those with fewer than 10 partners. Among merchant seamen in Norway (20), the prevalence of HBV serologic markers was 9%. Men with frequent casual sexual contacts, however, had a prevalence of 15% compared with 8% in men with no or infrequent casual contacts.

Table I Prevalence of HBV infection in heterosexuals by amount of recent sexual activity

Population/Activity		HBV Markers	Reference	(Country)
STD	< 3 partners	1%	16	(UK)
	≥ 3 partners	18%		
STD	< 5 partners	6%	17	(USA)
	≥ 5 partners	21%		
Students	< 3 partners	2%	17	(USA)
	≥ 3 partners	14%		

Table II Prevalence of HBV infection in heterosexuals by amount of lifetime sexual activity

Population/Activity		HBV Markers	Reference	(Country)
STD	≤ 5 partners	9%	19	(UK)
	> 5 partners	30%		
STD	< 50 partners	5%	17	(USA)
	≥ 50 partners	20%		
Students	< 10 partners	2%	17	(USA)
	≥ 10 partners	7%		
Merchant Seamen			20	(Norway)
	0-few casual contacts	8%		
	Frequent casual contacts	15%		

Studies among female prostitutes have also been done to examine the risk of HBV infection as a result of sexual activity (Table III). In several of these studies, when prostitutes were compared with blood donors or other 'low risk' women from the general population, the prostitutes were found to have a prevalence of HBV infection 2 to 4 fold higher than the controls (21-24). Specific risk factors found to be associated with an increased risk of HBV infection included duration of prostitution and history of other STDs. Risk of infection was associated with increasing numbers of partners in only one study (21). One other study in a prostitute population failed to find a difference in the prevalence of HBV infection between the prostitutes and three control groups (25); however, the persons selected as controls had other risk factors for HBV infection, such as health care occupation and institutionalization.

An association between HBV infection and a history of other STDs has been found in other populations. Among heterosexual men attending an STD clinic in Copenhagen, the overall prevalence of HBV infection was 12% (28). Men with a previous history of STDs, however, had an HBV prevalence rate as high as 50%. Mele et al. examined a number of partners in the preceding year and previous history of STDs in men and women attending an STD clinic in Italy (27). This study found an increased risk of HBV infection to be associated with seropositivity for antibody to herpes simplex virus type 2. Two of the studies in other populations mentioned above that found an association between HBV infection and number of recent or lifetime partners also found an association between HBV infection and history of other STDs (17,19).

Table III Prevalence of HBV infection in heterosexual women with different sexual behaviors

Population	HBV Markers	Factors	Reference	(Country)
Prostitutes	61%	Duration	24	(Greece)
Pregnant Women	28%			
Prostitutes	25%		25	(Columbia)
Clinic patients	21%			
Prisoners	33%			
Nuns	33%			
Prostitutes	33%	Duration	22	(FRG)
Blood donors	10%	Other STDs		
Nuns	14%			
Prostitutes	84%	Other STDs	21	(Spain)
General population	24%	No. partners		

Of particular interest in assessing the role of sexual activity in the transmission of HBV between heterosexuals are the results of two population based studies conducted in the United States. One of these was a seroepidemiologic survey of a random sample of households in Belle Glade, Florida, which provided the opportunity to evaluate risk factors for HBV infection in a racially mixed community (28). The overall prevalence of HBV infection was 26%, higher than the 5% reported in the United States general population. Few persons were found to have other risk factors for HBV infection including homosexual activity and parenteral drug use, and these were excluded from the analysis. Risk factors found to be associated with HBV infection among the adults in this community were a positive test for syphilis and having 2 or more lifetime sexual partners, each of which was associated with a 2- to 3-fold increased risk in both men and women. The second study reported results from a serologic survey of a probability sample of the United States population (National Health and Nutrition Examination Survey [NHANES II]) conducted between 1976 and 1980 (29). The prevalence of HBV infection among blacks was almost 5 times higher than among whites (14% vs. 3%), and both black race and seropositivity for syphilis were found to be independently associated with HBV seropositivity; data on number of sexual partners were not obtained.

Prevention of sexually transmitted HBV infections

Prevention of hepatitis B is easily accomplished through the use of hepatitis B vaccine given before exposure to infection. Unfortunately, hepatitis B vaccine has not been widely used for the prevention of sexually transmitted HBV infection despite long-standing recommendations that homosexually active men, persons with multiple sexual partners, or those with multiple episodes of sexually transmitted diseases be immunized (2). There are many reasons for the lack of hepatitis B vaccine use. The most important appears to be a lack of knowledge on the part of patients and health care providers that hepatitis B is a sexually transmitted disease; especially that it can be acquired by heterosexual activity. A study done in 1985 to determine the knowledge and practices of physicians concerning the prevention of hepatitis B, showed that only 45% knew homosexual activity was a risk factor for HBV infection or that sexual contacts of patients with hepatitis B were at risk of infection; only 10% were aware that heterosexual activity with multiple partners was a risk factor (CDC, unpublished data).

Most of the populations with high rates of infection are not aware of their risk or do not become aware of their risk until they have become infected, making control of the disease very difficult in these groups. In addition, approximately 30% of patients with hepatitis B have no identifiable source of infection (3), placing them out of reach of a strategy that targets only high risk groups. As the cost of hepatitis B vaccine decreases, there is a greater likelihood that universal immunization of infants or adolescents will become a viable means of controlling hepatitis B. In the meantime, it is important to specifically identify patients at risk of infection and provide either pre-exposure or post-exposure prophylaxis for hepatitis B.

References

1. Maynard JE, Kane MA, Alter MJ, et al (1988) In: Zuckerman AJ, ed. Viral Hepatitis and Liver Disease. New York, NY: Alan R. Liss, Inc, p. 967.
2. Centers for Disease Control (1990) MMWR 39 (No. RR-1).
3. Alter MJ, Hadler SC, Margolis HS, et al (1990) JAMA 263: 1218.
4. Koff RS, Slavin MM, Connelly LJD, et al (1977) Gastroenterology 72: 297.
5. Peters CJ, Purcell RH, Lander JJ, et al (1976) J Infect Dis 134: 218.
6. Redeker AG, Mosley JW, Gocke DJ, et al (1975) N Engl J Med 193: 1055.
7. Bernier RH, Sampliner R, Gerety R, et al (1982) Am J Epidemiol 116: 199.
8. Heathcote J, Gateau PH, Sherlock S (1974) Lancet 2: 370.
9. Irwin GR, Allen AM, Bancroft WH, et al (1974) JAMA 227: 1012.
10. Szmuness W, Harley EJ, Prince AM (1975) Am J Med Sci 270: 293.
11. Szmuness W, Prince AM, Hirsch RL, et al (1973) N Eng J Med 289: 1162.
12. Wright RA (1975) JAMA 232: 717.
13. Clee WB, Hunter PR (1987) Brit Med J 295: 530.
14. Heathcote J, Sherlock S (1973) Lancet 1: 1468.
15. Papaevangelou G, Roumeliofou-Karayannis A, Tassopoulos N, et al (1983) J Infect Dis 147: 987.
16. Fulford KWM, Dane DS (1973) Lancet 1: 1470.
17. Alter MJ, Ahtone J, Weisfuse I, et al (1988) JAMA 256: 1307.
18. Alter MJ, Coleman PJ, Alexander WJ, et al (1989) JAMA 262: 1201.
19. Baddour LM, Bucak VA, Somes G, et al (1988) Sex Transm Dis 15: 174.
20. Siebke JC, Wessel N, Kvandal P, et al (1989) Infection 17: 77.

21. Caballero LR, Caballero CR, Caballero IR, et al (1987) Epidem Inf 99: 767.
22. Frosner GG, Buchholz HM, Gerth HJ (1975) Am J Epidemiol 102: 241.
23. Kaklamani E, Kyriakidou A, Trichopoulos D, et al (1980) J Hyg Camb 84: 257.
24. Papaevangelou G, Trichopoulos D, Kremastinou T, et al (1974) Brit Med J 2: 256.
25. Adam E, Hollinger B, Melnick JL, et al (1974) J Infect Dis 129: 317.
26. Hentzer B, Skinhoj P, Hoybye G, et al (1980) Scand J Infect Dis 12: 245.
27. Mele A, Franco E, Caprilli F, et al (1988) Eur J Epidemiol 4: 488.
28. Rosenblum LS, Hadler SC, Castro KG, et al (1990) J Infect Dis 161: 407.
29. McQuillan GM, Townsend TR, Fields HA, et al (1989) Am J Med 87(suppl 3A): 5S.

Hepatitis B: A sexually transmitted disease in heterosexuals.
P. Piot and F.E. Andre, editors

The importance of heterosexual transmission of hepatitis B in Italy

P. PASQUINI, A. MELE, M.A. STAZI

Istituto Superiore di Sanità, Rome, Italy

Introduction

Viral hepatitis is one of the most important public health problems in Italy. Every year 9000 Italians die from liver cirrhosis and hepatocellular carcinoma attributable to hepatitis B infection (1); this is a consequence of the wide exposure of the Italian population to HBV during the past decades and of the early acquisition of the infection during life, often in childhood, due to intrafamilial person to person transmission, the most common mode of transmission in Italy until recent years (2). This picture, as suggested by national age-type-specific notification rates (3) and by serologic data (4-6), is rapidly changing; the age of maximum incidence of hepatitis B in Italy is now around adolescence reflecting mostly sexual exposure (1, 3). Sexual transmission of hepatitis B virus has long been recognized (7-13); in particular homosexuals are regarded as a group at high risk of acquiring hepatitis B (14-17), but prostitutes are also a high risk group (18, 19), and more recently the importance of heterosexual activity in the transmission of hepatitis B has been recognized (20-27).

In order to assess in quantitative terms the risk associated with heterosexual exposure in the Italian population, data from the nationwide type-specific surveillance of acute hepatitis cases in Italy (SEIEVA) and preliminary data from a case-control study on hepatitis B and non-A, non-B hepatitis in Naples (Italy), were used.

Study population and methods

SEIEVA

The nationwide type-specific surveillance system for acute viral hepatitis (SEIEVA) was established in Italy in 1984 by the Istituto Superiore di Sanità (the Italian National Institute of Health). It is based on 153 Health Departments scattered all over the country, covering 27% of the Italian population. The principal aims of SEIEVA are to promote local investigations and control for acute viral hepatitis cases, describe distribution of disease by time, space and persons, establish priorities for prevention and evaluate the impact of prevention programmes. The data reported in this paper refer to the years 1985-1989; no changes in the notification system were introduced in Italy in the period considered; the vast majority of acute hepatitis cases in Italy are hospitalized and virtually all hospitalized cases are notified; no changes in the hospitalized/non-hospitalized ratio have been reported in Italy over the last 4 years.

On receipt of each notified case of acute viral hepatitis, public health departments contact hospitals or medical practitioners to collect the results of serological tests for hepatitis B surface antigen (HBsAg) and hepatitis A IgM (IgM anti-HAV). Test results are recorded weekly on a line listing of cases which also records age, sex and week of onset of each case. Following notification, each case is interviewed by a public health doctor or inspector using a standard questionnaire. Both weekly line listing of cases and questionnaires are forwarded to the study center at the Istituto Superiore di Sanità.

A hepatitis A case was defined as a subject with an acute hepatitis and with IgM anti-HAV; hepatitis B case as a subject with HBsAg and without IgM anti-HAV; patients without both IgM anti-HAV and HBsAg were defined as hepatitis Non-A,Non-B cases. A subject without (or not tested) HBsAg and not tested (or without) IgM anti-HAV was an unspecified case.

Hepatitis A and hepatitis B acute cases were observed in the same geographical areas during the same periods and in the same hospitals. They are comparable as far as socio-economic status is concerned. Hepatitis A cases were used as controls providing estimates of proportion of exposure to blood transfusion, hospitalization, number of sexual partners, etc. among non-hepatitis B cases.

Naples Case-Control Study

This is an ongoing hospital-based case-control study on the incident of cases of A, B and non-A, non-B hepatitis, in Naples coordinated by the Istituto Superiore di Sanità since November 1987. The area of Naples is endemic for viral hepatitis; it is served by one single hospital for infectious diseases, and is covered by the SEIEVA network. The principal objective of the study is to estimate the relative and attributable risk for the disease, associated with transfusion, drug abuse, other parenteral exposures, sexual behavior and household contact with a HBsAg carrier.

Case definition

A hepatitis B case was defined as a patient with acute viral hepatitis resident in Naples and province, with presence in serum sample of HBsAg and of antibodies of hepatitis B core antigen (anti-HBc).

Controls are defined as follows:

1) patients resident in Naples or province, attending infectious diseases clinics, participating to the study and dismissed after onset of the following infectious diseases no more than 15 days before the date of admission: pertussis, measles, pneumonia, mumps, meningitis, rickettsia, herpetic stomatitis, erysipelas, brucellosis, non-mononucleotic angina;
2) patients resident in Naples and province, attending the neurosurgery and ENT departments of the pediatric hospital 'Santobono' for the following diseases: laryngospasm, otorrhea, nose fracture, otitis media, foreign body, cyst, cleft palate;
3) patients resident in Naples and province, 12 years old or more, admitted to 'Cardarelli' hospital in traumatology, orthopedics and surgery divisions, for accidents, surgical interventions for hernia and appendicitis.

A standard precoded questionnaire was used, to collect information on:

1) demographic variables: age, sex, education, type of work;
2) presence of chronic liver disease;
3) drug and alcohol consumption;

4) principal risk factors for hepatitis transmitted by parenteral as well as fecal-oral route.

Serological and statistical techniques

IgM anti-HAV, HBsAg and IgM anti-HBc are detected by ELISA.

Statistical analysis was based on the Mantel-Haenszel procedure for adjusting odds ratios (28); the Miettinen method was used for calculating confidence limits (29).

A multiple logistic function was also used (30) and the multiple adjusted odds ratios, corresponding to the estimated ß coefficients of the logistic function, derived (31).

Results

A total of 2133 acute hepatitis cases 15 years old and older (1414 males and 719 females) classified by the SEIEVA system as hepatitis B were investigated, and information on their heterosexual exposure collected and compared with that of 933 controls.

The heterosexual exposure of 64 hepatitis B cases 15 years old and older was compared with that of 106 controls in the Naples case-control study.

Using the data of the nationwide surveillance system, the age adjusted Mantel-Haenszel Odds Ratio estimating the risk associated with exposure to two or more heterosexual partners as compared to one or none, is 2.2 (1.6-2.9) for males (Table I) and 2.7 (1.2-6.2) for females (Table II); using the data of the case-control study it is 3.9 (1.5-10.3) for males 15-24 years of age (Table III), while no evidence of the association appears in the case-control data for females and older males.

Table I Hepatitis B and heterosexual exposure SEIEVA National Data – Italy

Males

No. of heterosexual partners in previous year.

	2 or more	0-1	
HBV cases	566	848	1414
Controls	68	220	288
	634	1068	1702

$O.R_{MH} = 2.2$ (1.6-2.9)

Multiple adjustment by a logistic function slightly reduces the strength of the association: 1.5 (1.2-1.8) for males and 2.0 (1.1-3.6) for females (Table IV).

For subjects under 25, in the SEIEVA data we observed a trend: the risk of hepatitis B increases with the number of heterosexual partners in the previous year (Table V).

Table II Hepatitis B and heterosexual exposure SEIEVA National Data – Italy

Females

No. of heterosexual partners in previous year.

	2 or more	0-1	
HBV cases	80	639	719
Controls	7	164	171
	87	803	890

$OR._{MH} = 2.7\ (1.2\text{-}6.2)$

Table III Hepatitis B and heterosexual exposure preliminary data from Naples – case-control study

Males under 25

No. of heterosexual partners in previous year

	2 or more	0-1	
HBV cases	15	31	46
Controls	8	65	73
	23	96	119

OR = 3.9 (1.5-10.3)

Table IV SEIEVA National Data – Italy – risk of Hepatitis B associated to heterosexual exposures* after multiple adjustment**

Multiple logistic function ß coefficients		Corresponding Mantel Haenszel multiple adjusted odds ratios	
Males	0.407	1.5	(1.2-1.8)
Females	0.681	2.0	(1.1-3.6)

* Heterosexual exposure: 2 or more partners versus 0-1, in previous year.

** Multiple adjustment. For males: age, use of drugs, area of residence, hospital, blood transfusion, surgery, dentist, barber; for females: age, use of drugs.

Table V Hepatitis B and heterosexual transmission – SEIEVA National Data – Italy

Risk of hepatitis by no. heterosexual partners (odds ratios)

No. of partners in previous year		0-1	2-3	4-5	6 or more
Age	15-24	1	1.9	2.0	2.4
	25 and over	1	3.0	1.6	2.0

Discussion

The incidence of notified cases of viral hepatitis has been decreasing in Italy since 1970 (1). We have evidence that this phenomenon affected all types of hepatitis and that the age specific incidence rates are changing (1, 3). In particular the age of maximum incidence of hepatitis B, which used to be in the age group 0-14, is now in the age group 15-24. In 1988 this rate was 22/100,000 in the age group 15-24 and 2/100,000 in the age group 0-14 (Table VI). Recent seroepidemiological evidence confirms this observation (4, 5, 7).

Table VI Incidence rates per 100,000 Hepatitis B cases in Italy per year and age. SEIEVA

Years	Age	Incidence rates	Years	Age	Incidence rates
	0-14	6		0-14	3
1985	15-24	41	1986	15-24	35
	25 >	7		25 >	9
	TOTAL	12		TOTAL	12
	0-14	2		0-14	2
1987	15-24	31	1988	15-24	22
	25 >	8		25 >	5
	TOTAL	10		TOTAL	7

We believe that the main determinants of this reduction are not medical but rather socio-demographic in nature. Particularly important in this regard is probably the reduction of family size, a phenomenon observed in Italy over the last few decades as a consequence of the transformation of the Italian society from mostly agricultural to a fully industrial one; many disincentives to have babies (urbanization and related housing problems, the job of the mother, financial considerations, etc.) determined a decrease of the Italian national birth rate which is now one of the lowest in the world. The reduced number of children in a single family and the tendency of families to be 'nuclear' reduced the 'force of infection' and the 'reproduction rate' (32) of hepatitis B affecting its dynamics in the Italian population. The observed changes in the age of maximum incidence of infection suggest that the relative importance of sexual activity is becoming greater in the transmission of hepatitis B infection in Italy. Data presented in this paper confirm that heterosexual exposure in particular is a determinant of hepatitis B incidence particularly in the 15-24 age group. In a recent study (33) we reported that household or sexual exposure might account for as much as 18% of the total hepatitis B infection in Italy (Table VI). We used hepatitis A cases as controls of hepatitis B cases in the SEIEVA data because in case-control studies comparability is more important than representativeness and in our study both hepatitis types were identified through the same surveillance system in the same areas. Should hepatitis A and B share some risk factors, our odds ratios would be underestimated.

As a consequence of the lower and later exposure in life, among the Italian population, we will probably see a reduction of liver cirrhosis and hepatocarcinoma in the next decades in Italy, even in the absence of any intervention. But, if we want to reinforce this trend we have to adopt rational immunization strategies such as vaccination of teenagers and other categories with high sexual exposure; it cannot be overemphasized that all other non-immunologic preventive measures, such as appropriate health information, promotion of condom use, etc. (33, 34) retain all their importance and, moreover, being non-'vertical' interventions, they are effective not only on hepatitis B, but on all other sexually transmitted diseases.

Table VII Proportion of all Hepatitis B cases attributable to particular risk factors. SEIEVA 1985-1987

Risk factors	Estimated exposure prevalence in population (%)	Attributable risk (%)
Surgical intervention	3	4
Hospitalization	14	11
Other percutaneous exposure	4	4
Barber shop shaving	2	2
Dental therapy	13	9
I. V. drug abuse	0.08	0.4
Household or sexual contact with HBsAg positive carrier	2.6	18

From: Mele A, Stazi AM, Gill ON, Pasquini P (1990) Prevention of hepatitis B in Italy: lessons from surveillance of type-specific acute viral hepatitis. Epidemiol Infect 104: 135-141.

References

1. Mele A, Stroffolini T, Ferrigno L et al (1989) SEIEVA. Sistema Epidemiologico Integrato dell'Epatite Virale Acuta. Campagna Vaccinale Antiepatite B in Italia. Istituto Superiore di Sanità, Rapporto ISTISAN 89/40, Roma, p. 1.
2. Dardanoni L, Mele A, Polizzi MC (1988) Ann Ist Super Sanità 24: 235.
3. Mele A, Stazi MA, Corona R, et al. Decline of incidence of A, B and Non-A,Non-B hepatitis in Italy. Results of four years surveillance (1985-1988) (Paper in preparation).
4. D'Argenio P, Esposito D, Mele A et al. Decline in the exposure to hepatitis A and B infections in children in Naples, Italy. Public Health (in press).
5. Stroffolini T, Franco E, Romano G et al. Hepatitis B virus infection in children in Sardinia, Italy. Eur J Epidemiol (in press).
6. Stroffolini T, Craxi A, Gianmarco A et al. Hepatitis B virus infection in children in Palermo, Italy. (submitted for publication).
7. Vahrman J (1970) Lancet 2: 774.
8. Mersch T, Melnick JL, Goyal RK et al (1971). N Engl J Med 285: 1363.
9. Vahrman J (1973) Lancet 2: 157.
10. Fulford KWM (1973) Lancet 1: 1470.
11. Heathcote J, Gateau P, Scherlock S (1974) Lancet 2: 370.
12. Szmuness W, Much M, Prince A et al (1975) Ann Intern Med 83: 489.
13. Peters C, Purcell R, Lander J, Johnson K (1976) J Infect Dis 134: 218.

14. Dietzman DE, Harnisch JP, Ray CG, Alexander ER, Holmes KK (1977) JAMA 238: 2625.
15. Fawaz KA, Matloff DS (1981) Gastroenterology 81: 537.
16. Hansfield HH (1981) AJPH 71: 989.
17. Schereeder MT, Thompson SE, Hadler SC et al (1982) J Infect Dis 146: 7.
18. Goh CL, Kamarudin A, Chan SH, Rajan VS (1985) Genitourin Med 61: 127.
19. Goh CL, Rajan VS, Chan SH, Kamarudin A (1986) Int J Epidemiol 15: 112.
20. Papaevangelou G, Roumeliotou-Karayannis A, Tassopolous N, Kolaitis N, Stathopoulou P (1983) J Infect Dis 147: 987.
21. Alter MJ, Ahotone J, Weisfuse I, Starko K, Vacalis DT, Maynard JE (1986) JAMA 256: 1307.
22. Heun E, Whitworth B, Vogt R et al (1987) JAMA 257: 314.
23. Baddour LM, Bucak VA, Somes G, Hudson R (1988) Sexually Transmitted Diseases 15: 174.
24. Alter MJ, Coleman PJ, Alexander WJ et al (1989) JAMA 262: 1201.
25. C.D.C. US Department of Health and Human Services (1988) MMWR 37: 429.
26. Kane MA, Alter MJ, Hadler SC, Margolis HS (1989) Am J Med 87(suppl 3A): 11S.
27. Mele A, Franco E, Caprilli G, et al (1988) Eur J Epidemiol 4: 488.
28. Mantel N, Haenszel W (1959) J Natl Cancer Inst 22: 719.
29. Miettinen OS (1974) Am J Epidemiol 100: 515.
30. Schelesselman JJ (1982) Case-control studies. Design conduct analysis. Monographs in Epidemiology. Oxford University Press, New York.
31. Kahn HA, Sempos CT (1989) Statistical Methods in Epidemiology. Oxford University Press, New York.
32. Pasquini P, Delimar N, Kosicek M, De Blasio R, Raschetti R, Cvjetanovic B (1987) Eur J Epidemiol 3: 19.
33. Mele A, Stazi MA, Gill ON, Pasquini P and SEIEVA collaborating group (1990) Epidemiol Infect 104: 135.
34. Pasquini P (1988) Epidemiologia e Prevenzione 37: 60.

HBV MARKERS IN HETEROSEXUALS AND STD PATIENTS

© 1990 Elsevier Science Publishers B.V. (Biomedical Division)
Hepatitis B: A sexually transmitted disease in heterosexuals.
P. Piot and F.E. Andre, editors

Heterosexual transmission of hepatitis B: data from Greece

GEORGE PAPAEVANGELOU AND ANASTASIA ROUMELIOTOU

National Center for Viral Hepatitis, Athens School of Hygiene, P.O. Box 140 85, Athens, Greece

Introduction

The discovery of the hepatitis B surface antigen (HBsAg) of the hepatitis B virus (HBV) gave the opportunity for the development of diagnostic assays that permitted the implementation of seroepidemiological surveys. Thus the pattern of the disease caused by HBV, its modes of transmission and the population groups at risk were determined. The different patterns of transmission and maintenance of HBV in different areas and populations were revealed. It was proved that in developing countries HBV infection occurs perinatally or very early in life, whereas in developed countries most infections occur in young adults with particular transmission patterns that dominate in different areas, even among the same population, depending on certain specific environmental and behavioral characteristics. Several studies estimated the importance of the various risk factors involved in the transmission of HBV and thus contributed to the control of the disease, especially in countries like Greece where HBV infection is a major public health problem (1).

Sexual transmission

Epidemiological surveys indicated very soon the patterns of HBV spread and determined groups at risk. The implementation of a National Vaccination Program (2) in polytransfused and renal dialysis patients, in drug addicts and in health care personnel limited the spread of HBV in these groups.

The obligatory screening of blood donors also dramatically reduced the incidence of post transfusion hepatitis B (3). However the morbidity and mortality of HBV disease in the general public remained high. It is estimated that there are in Greece about 250,000 HBsAg chronic carriers who are the source of HBV infection. The pattern of the spread of HBV in the general public (4) and the prevalence of HBV markers in sexually active persons, such as prostitutes (5), homosexuals (6) and STD patients support the significant role of sexual transmission of HBV in Greece.

Table I shows the prevalence of HBV infections in a random sample of the general population aged from 18 to 45 years old. The prevalence of HBV markers were more than two times higher in persons aged more than 20 years compared to those aged less than 20 years old, probably suggesting the spread of HBV through sexual intercourse.

Table I Prevalence of HBV markers in a random sample of general population and in sexual partners of chronic carriers by age

Age (years)	General population			Sexual partners of HBsAg carriers		
	No. examined	No. positive	%	No. examined	No. positive	%
<20	26	3	11.5	2	0	0
20-24	98	21	21.4	17	4	23.5
25-29	117	25	21.4	24	7	29.2
30-34	47	12	25.5	18	6	33.3
35+	41	13	31.7	10	9	90.0
Total	329	74	22.5	71	26	36.6

A very high prevalence of HBV infections has been detected in female prostitutes of the Greater Athens Area (Table II), which is increasing with age and with duration of professional activity (5).

Greek homosexual men have also a high frequency of HBV infections. The frequency was found higher among anti-HIV positives (73.3%) than anti-HIV negatives (52.2%). Anti-HIV positive homosexuals reported a higher number of sexual contacts per month, a higher frequency of syphilis and gonorrhea and a lower frequency of condom use (6) suggesting that sexual practices and behaviors are factors determining the spread of HBV. This is also supported by the high spread of HBV among STD patients.

Table II Prevalence of HBV markers in female prostitutes by age

Age (years)	No. examined	HBV infected	
		No.	%
20-24	18	11	61.1
25-29	73	36	49.3
30-34	57	36	63.2
> 35	138	93	67.4
Total	293	179	61.1

Heterosexual transmission

Retrospective and prospective data from sexual partners of HBV infected persons proved that heterosexual transmission is one of the most important routes of HBV transmission in adults.

Retrospective data

The importance of heterosexual transmission of HBV in Greece was confirmed from the increased prevalence of HBV markers in heterosexual partners of chronic HBsAg carriers (4) compared to the general population (Table I). It was supported also by the higher frequency of chronic carriers among heterosexual partners af acute hepatitis B patients (28.4%) (7) compared to the frequency among heterosexual partners of acute hepatitis A (5.8%) and non A-non B patients (6.6%) (Table III).

Table III Frequency of HBsAg carriers among heterosexual partners of patients with acute hepatitis

type of hepatitis	No. of patients	No. of carrier partners	Percent (%)
A	69	4	5.8
B	415	118	28.4
non A-non B	106	7	6.6

The HBsAg positive heterosexual partners of acute hepatitis B patients were considered as the source of infection for the patients, since no other risk factors were reported (8). The carrier rate was higher in male heterosexual partners (47.5%) than in female partners (12.9%) of acute hepatitis B patients (Table IV) suggesting more efficient transmisson from males to females than from females to males, as is the case for all other sexually transmitted diseases.

Table IV The carriage of hepatitis B surface antigen (HBsAg) by sex in sexual partners and control subjects in Greece

Sex of index case	Sexual partners			Controls		
	No. examined	HBsAg positive	%	No. examined	HBsAg positive	%
Male	40	19	47.5	517	17	3.3
Female	62	8	12.9	1271	20	1.6
Total	102	27	26.5	1788	37	2.1

The HBsAg positive partners were more frequently HBsAg-positive (8) than control carriers found through blood donor screening (Table V). Our data showed that mainly HBeAg but also anti-HBe positive carriers may transmit the virus to their sexual partners.

HBV DNA should be considered as a better marker of contagiousness. According to our data, HBV DNA was detected in 96.9% of the HBeAg positive and in 41% of the anti-HBe positive carriers who were the source of infection to their heterosexual partners. However it was detected in only 11.6% of carriers whose heterosexual partners showed no serological findings of recent or past HBV infection (9).

Table V The frequency of indications of increased contagiousness of sexual partners and control subjects who are carriers of hepatitis B surface antigen

Criteria	Sexual partners (%)	Control subjects (%)
SGPT >40 IU	48.1	5.4
HBeAg	29.6	2.6
Anti-HBe	70.4	97.3

Prospective data

Follow up of 45 susceptible-to-HBV heterosexual partners of 45 chronic hepatitis B carriers (median follow up 15 months) showed that 3 of them were infected by HBV. Two of them developed clinical and another one subclinical acute hepatitis B (4).

Susceptible-to-HBV heterosexual partners of acute hepatitis B patients were also prospectively examined (10). Seventy one of them were followed up for nine months. They were clinically examined and serologically tested for HBV markers. During the follow up period 18.3% of them were infected by HBV (7.0% clinically and 11.3% subclinically) (Table VI).

Table VI Attack rate in susceptible to HBV spouses of acute Hepatitis B patients by sex

Sex of spouse	No. examined	No. infected	%
Male	27	3	11.5
Female	44	10	22.7
Total	71	13	18.3

The attack rate of female spouses (22.7%) was higher than that of male spouses (11.5%) and agreed very well with our retrospective data suggesting the greater efficiency of male to female transmission.

We conclude that: 1. Heterosexual transmission of HBV should be considered as the most important route of HBV infection among Greek adults. 2. Male to female transmission is more efficient than female to male. 3. HBV DNA should be considered as a better marker of infectivity than HBeAg/anti HBe status.

References

1. Papaevangelou G, Kyriakidou A, Vissoulis C, Trichopoulos D (1976) J Hyg (Camb) 76: 229.
2. Papaevangelou G In Viral Hepatitis and Liver Diseases. Proceedings of the 1984 International Symposium on Viral Hepatitis. Ed. Vyas G, Dienstang J, Grune and Stratton Orlando Florida pp 587.

3. Papaevangelou G, (1980) Biblithca haematol. 46: 15.
4. Stathopoulou-Denediou P. (1984) Need for HBV screening before marriage. Medical School University of Athens. Thesis..
5. Papaevangelou G, Trichopoulos D, Kremastinou T, Papoutsakis G. BMJ 1: 256: 258, (1974).
6. Papaevangelou G, Kallinikos G, Roumeliotou A, Ktenas E, Kotsianopoulou M (1990). Prevalence of HIV infections in Greek homosexuals. A five year study (submitted for publication).
7. Papaevangelou G, Tassopoulos N, Roumeliotou-Karayannis A, Richardson C (1985) J Inf. Dis 152: 231.
8. Papaevangelou G, Roumeliotou-Karayannis A, Tassopoulos N, Kalaitis N, Stathopoulou P. (1983) J Infec Dis 147: 987.
9. Tassopoulos N, Papaevangelou G, Roumeliotou-Karayannis A, Ticehurst J, Feinstone S, Purcell R. (1987) Am J Epid 126: 587.
10. Roumeliotou-Karayannis A, Papaevangelou G, Tassopoulos N, Richardson C, Krugman S. (1985) Vaccine 3: 31.

© 1990 Elsevier Science Publishers B.V. (Biomedical Division)
Hepatitis B: A sexually transmitted disease in heterosexuals.
P. Piot and F.E. Andre, editors

Sexual transmission of hepatitis viruses

Georg Hess, Anja Massing, Siegbert Rossol, Rita Voth, Ralf Clemens, Hans Schütt, Karl Hermann Meyer zum Büschenfelde

I. Medical Department and Blood Bank, Johannes Gutenberg University, Mainz, Langenbeckstraße 1, 6500 Mainz, F. R. G.

Introduction

Recently a new virus termed hepatitis C virus (HCV) which is responsible for the majority of parenterally transmitted cases of non A, non B hepatitis has been identified and partially characterized (1). Epidemiological studies indicate, that this type of hepatitis is predominantly transmitted by parenteral exposure e.g. blood transfusion or illicit intravenous drug abuse (2). The recent detection of the hepatitis C virus enabled the development of a test to detect antibodies to HCV (anti-HCV) (1,3). Preliminary experience indicates that anti-HCV is frequently present in individuals with chronic non A, non B hepatitis and parenteral exposure to blood and blood products. However, anti-HCV is frequently positive in patients who are diagnosed as having chronic non A, non B hepatitis by exclusion of other causes of chronic hepatitis and who have had no perceivable parenteral exposure (3-7).

One potential mode of HCV infection might be sexual transmission (4). Sexual transmission of type B hepatitis (8,9) has already been demonstrated and transmission of type A hepatitis has been established in case of homosexual activity (10).

The objective of the present epidemiological study was to determine the prevalence of hepatitis A, B and C infection in patients with sexually transmitted diseases (STD) and to compare the results with those in a control (blood donors) group.

Patients and methods

Subjects

Sera of 191 heterosexual patients with sexually transmitted diseases (STD) were analysed, 105 males and 86 females (mean age 39.1 years, range 17-73 years). 39 presented with syphilis, 5 with condylomata acuminata, 6 with gonorrhoea and 141 with recurrent genital herpes. As control sera of 390 blood donors (mean age 36.2 years, range 18-61 years) were analysed. They were random consecutive blood donors from the blood bank in Mainz, FRG. Routine syphilis serology was positive in 9 of the blood donors.

Sera were kept at -20°C until analysed.

The study was approved by a local ethical review committee and performed according to the Declaration of Helsinki.

Tests
Sera were tested for antibodies to hepatitis A virus (anti-HAV) and antibodies to hepatitis B core antigen (anti-HBc) by commercial tests (Abbott Laboratories, Chicago, Illinois, USA).

Sera positive for anti-HBc were also analysed for hepatitis B surface antigen (HBsAg) and antibodies to HBsAg (anti-HBs) by commercial tests (Abbott Laboratories).

Antibodies to HCV (anti-HCV) were tested by a newly developed enzyme immunoassay (Ortho Diagnostics Neckargemünd, FRG) (1,3).

All tests were done twice. In case of any discrepancy sera were reanalysed.

Statistics
The age distribution in the two groups was compared by the Wilcoxon-test. For comparing the prevalence of the 3 types of hepatitis in the different groups (STD, blood donors), Chi-square tests were used. Because of the small sample size in patients positive for HBsAg or anti-HBs, these data were compared by means of Fisher's exact test.

The relation between different types of hepatitis and between hepatitis B and different STD was examined by Chi-square tests.

Results

Both groups, patients with STD and blood donors (representing a sample of the normal population as control) were comparable for age and age distribution.

Table I shows the prevalence of hepatitis viruses A, B and C in STD patients and blood donors.

The prevalence of hepatitis B as measured by anti-HBc was significantly higher in STD patients when compared to blood donors ($p < 0.001$). Anti-HBs was present in 38/59 (64.4%) anti-HBc positive STD patients and in 14/16 (87.5%) blood donors positive for anti-HBc. Of the 9 blood donors who were positive for syphilis serology, 2 had anti-HBc but neither of them was positive for HBsAg or anti-HBs.

The percentage of patients with antibodies to the hepatitis C virus (anti-HCV) was also significantly higher in STD patients than in blood donors ($p < 0.001$, Table I).

Table I Hepatitis A, B and C viruses in blood donors and individuals with sexually transmitted diseases

	STD patients	Blood donors	
anti-HBc	59/191 (30.9%)	16/390 (4.1%)	$p < 0.001$
HBsAg	11/ 59 (18.6%)	0/ 16 (0%)	$p = 0.058$ (n.s.)*
anti-HBs	38/ 59 (64.4%)	14/ 16 (87.5%)	$p = 0.07$ (n.s.)*
anti-HCV	9/191 (4.7%)	2/390 (0.51%)	$p < 0.001$
anti-HAV	90/191 (47.1%)	81/390 (20.8%)	$p < 0.0001$

* Fisher's exact test

Anti-HCV positivity was less frequent in recurrent genital herpes, although the prevalence of anti-HCV in this subgroup is still 4 to 5 times higher than in the control group.

Anti-HAV was more commonly found in STD patients than in blood donors, the difference in prevalence being statistically significant ($p < 0.0001$; Table I).

Table II specifies the prevalence of anti-HBc in the different types of STD. Previous or ongoing HBV infection was most frequently found in patients with syphilis, condylomata acuminata and gonorrhoea.

Table II Anti-HBc prevalence in different types of sexually transmitted diseases and in control group

	Anti HBc	positive
STD (total)	59/191	(30.9%)
- Syphilis	27/39	(69.2%)
- Condylomata accuminata	3/5	(60%)
- Gonorrhoea	3/6	(50%)
- Recurrent genital herpes	26/141	(18.4%)
Blood donors*	16/390	(0.4%)

* 9 blood donors were positive for syphilis serology with 2/9 being anti-HBc positive.

The individual data of all 9 anti-HCV positive STD patients are presented in Table III. The majority of these 9 patients was anti-HAV positive, and 5 of the 9 cases suffered from syphilis.

Table III Anti-HCV in nine STD patients: relation to other hepatitis viruses and underlying diseases

No.	Sex	Age (years)	Disease	anti-HBc	anti-HAV
1	F	34	HS	+	+
2	M	74	HS	+	+
3	M	53	Syph.	+	-
4	M	59	Syph.	+	+
5	F	27	HS	-	+
6	F	28	Syph.	-	-
7	F	29	Syph.	-	+
8	F	33	HS	-	+
9	M	49	Syph.	-	+

HS = recurrent genital herpes, F = female, M = male.

Table IV compares the presence of anti-HBc to the anti-HCV status in the total study population as well as in both groups. The figures indicating that hepatitis C infections are more common in individuals with previous exposure to the hepatitis B virus.

Table IV Anti-HCV in anti-HBc positive and anti-HBc negative subjects

	anti-HCV		
	Total	STD patients	Blood donors
anti-HBc positive	4/57 (5.3%)	4/59 (6.8%)	0/16 (0%)
anti-HBc negative	7/506 (1.4%)	5/132 (3.8%)	2/374 (0.5%)

$p < 0.05$.

The prevalence of anti-HAV is known to increase with age. This finding could be confirmed in our study. As the distribution of age was comparable in the STD group and in the group of blood donors, the 26% difference in anti-HAV prevalence cannot be attributed to a difference in age distribution.

Table V compares the anti-HAV status in the total study population and two sub-cohorts with the hepatitis B prevalence. In all groups a highly significant correlation between HAV and HBV infection could be detected.

Table V Anti-HAV in anti-HBc positive and anti-HBc negative subjects

	anti-HAV		
	Total	STD patients	Blood donors
anti-HBc positive	49/75 (65.3%)	37/59 (62.7%)	12/16 (75%)
anti-HBc negative	122/506 (24.1%)	53/132 (40.2%)	69/374 (18.4%)

$p < 0.005$; $p = 0.004$; $p < 0.05$.

Discussion

The present study analyses the prevalence of hepatitis A, B and C viruses in blood donors and in heterosexual patients suffering from sexually transmitted diseases. It confirms that type B hepatitis is frequently sexually transmitted (8-16). The high serum concentration of the hepatitis B virus in many HBsAg carriers enables transmission of the virus not only by sexual intercourse (8-17) but also, in contrast to the human immunodeficiency virus by other close contact, such as kissing. Thus, preventive measures such as the use of condoms might be effective in reducing transmission of HIV infection but only to some extent in the case of HBV infection.

The 30% prevalence of HBV infection in STD patients in this study is comparable to that established in long term health care workers (8). Limited studies indicate that sexual transmission represents the major mode of spread of type B hepatitis (8). However, this has so far not been adequately translated into prevention strategies. As it may be difficult to recognize and immunize sexually active and promiscuous individuals in time, only mass immunization programs in early childhood might be effective in significantly reducing or eradicating hepatitis B virus infection also in developed countries.

Until this goal has been successfully approached, it may be recommended that individuals at risk, namely those presenting with STD ought to be tested for anti-HBc. Those negative and susceptible for infection should be immunized against hepatitis B (19).

Anti-HCV testing in our STD population suggests that HCV is also sexually transmitted, but less efficiently than HBV, even if it is considered that approximately 50% of HCV infected patients recover and ultimately lose anti-HCV titers. This is most likely due to the lower HCV concentration in serum as compared with HBV. Studies in homosexuals and sexual partners of drug addicts confirm this assumption (4, our unpublished data). Effectiveness of sexual transmission of HCV is probably comparable to that of HIV with sexual intercourse, the only sexual practice at real risk. Condoms may therefore be effective in preventing the spread of HCV by sexual transmission.

Our data on sexual transmission of HAV are difficult to interpret. The post war generation in developed countries has a low prevalence of anti-HAV as confirmed in this study (20). HAV is usually acquired by travelling to developing countries. These countries are normally endemic for hepatitis A and also have frequently a high prevalence of hepatitis B virus carriers.

This could explain the surprisingly high correlation found in the presence of hepatitis A and hepatitis B serum markers. This might indicate as well that travellers to endemic areas (e.g. Asia, Africa) may require both active hepatitis B immunization and protection against hepatitis A. The latter is also of increasing significance as type A hepatitis runs a more severe course with increasing age. The development of an active immunization thus seems to be desirable in order to achieve long term hepatitis A protection, especially in view of increasing numbers of long distance travellers.

The high incidence of anti-HAV in STD patients compared to blood donors of the same age suggests an increased risk of HAV infection for this population and thus indicates the need for future hepatitis A prevention strategies in patients with STD. Whether the increased prevalence of HAV infection in patients with STD relates in fact to sexual transmission or to different behavior (e.g. frequent travelling) needs to be determined.

Acknowledgement

The work is part of the thesis of A. Massing. The authors appreciate the expert technical assistance of S. Schwickert and S. Jacobs.

References

1. Choo QL, Kuo G, Weiner AJ, Overby LR, Bradley DW, Houghton M (1989) Science 244: 359.
2. Alter H (1988) In: Viral hepatitis and Liver Disease, Alan R. Liss., Inc. New York, 537.
3. Kuo G, Choo QL, Alter H, Gitnick GL, Redeker AG, Purcell RH, Miyamura T, Dienstag JL, Alter MJ, Stevens CE, Tegtmeier GE, Bonino F, Colombo M, Lee WS, Kuo LC, Berger K, Shuster JR, Overby R, Bradley DW, Houghton M (1989) Science 244: 362.
4. Esteban JI, Viladomiu L, Roget M, Genesca J, Esteban R, Lopez-Talavera JC, Hernandez JM, Vargas V, Buti M (1989) Lancet 2: 294.
5. Van der Poel CL, Lelie PN, Choo QL, Ressink HW, Leentvaar-Kuypers A, Kuo G (1989) Lancet 5: 297.
6. Kühnl P, Seidl S, Stangel W, Beyer J, Sibrowski W, Flik J (1989) Lancet 2: 324 (Letter).
7. Roggendorf M, Deinhardt F, Rasshofer R, Eberle J, Hopf U, Möller B, Zachoval R, Pape G, Schramm W, Rommel F (1989) Lancet 5: 324 (Letter).

8. Maynard JE, Kane MA, Alter M, Hadler SC (1988) Control of hepatitis B by immunization: Global perspectives. Viral Hepatitis and Liver Disease, Alan R. Liss., Inc. New York, 967.
9. Alter M, Athone J, Weisfuse I, Starko K, Vacalis TD, Mayard JE (1986) JAMA 10 1307.
10. Hess G. Bienzle U, Slusarczyk J, Hannsson BG, Meyer zum Büschenfelde KH (1986) Liver 6: 13.
11. Christopher PJ, Mailer PT, Crewe EB, Murphy Am (1984) Aust NZ J Med 14: 491.
12. Hentzer B, Skinhoj P, Hojbye G, Nielsen AO, Kvorning SA, Faber V (1980) Scand J Infect Dis 12: 245.
13. Kryger P, Pedersen NJ, Mathiesen L, Nielsen OJ (1982) J Infect Dis 145: 23.
14. Adam E, Hollinger FB, Melnick JL, Duenas A, Rawls WE (1974) J Infect Dis 3: 317.
15. Papaevangelou G, Roumeliotou-Karayannis A, Tassopoulos N, Kolaitis N, Stahopoulou P (1983) J Infect Dis 6: 987.
16. Fagan EA, Davison F, Smith PM, Williams R (1986) Lancet 9: 538.
17. Gerety RJ (1988) In: Viral Hepatitis and Liver Disease, Alan R. Liss., Inc. New York, 1017.
18. Grady GF (1981) Sex Transmitt Dis 8: 344.
19. Ostrol DG, Behar PAC, Baker AE, Gremminger R, Krugman S, Stevens CE, Dull HB, Judson FN, Nylund TM, William DC, Darrow W, Holems KK, Thompson SE, Francis D, Reynolds GH (1982) Sex Transmitt. Dis 9: 151.
20. Flehmig B, Heinricy U, Pfister M (1989) Lancet 1: 1039.

© 1990 Elsevier Science Publishers B.V. (Biomedical Division)
Hepatitis B: A sexually transmitted disease in heterosexuals.
P. Piot and F.E. Andre, editors

Seroprevalence of hepatitis B virus infection in patients attending a genito-urinary medicine clinic

RJC GILSON*, A DE RUITER*, J WAITE+, C LOVEDAY+, G KELLY*, IVD WELLER*

*Academic Department of Genito-Urinary Medicine and +Department of Medical Microbiology, University College and Middlesex School of Medicine, London, U.K.

Introduction

There has been no recent published report of the prevalence and associated risk factors for hepatitis B virus (HBV) infection in a genito-urinary medicine (GUM) clinic population in the U.K. An early study from The Middlesex Hospital (1) showed an increased prevalence of markers of HBV infection amongst homosexual men which has been a consistent finding in later studies in the U.K., Europe, North America and Australia (2-8). Although the prevalence of HBV markers in heterosexuals attending clinics for sexually transmitted diseases has also been higher compared with hospital or blood donor populations, analysis of risk factors has yielded inconsistent results. This is despite the evidence of the increasing importance of heterosexual transmission of HBV infection in North America (9-10), although in the U.K. the proportion of reported cases of acute HBV infection attributable to heterosexual contact has not changed (11).

In this study, we have determined the prevalence and risk factors for HBV infection amongst a population of GUM clinic attenders surveyed in 1987. The earlier analysis of HIV prevalence, which was the initial aim of this survey, excluded patients participating in a prospective study of HIV infection, even if they were attending for another reason (12). In this analysis, these patients have been restored to the study population, the only exclusions being patients attending for routine follow-up of chronic HBV infection.

Methods

All patients attending the GUM clinic at the Middlesex Hospital during 4 weeks of November and December 1987 and having routine tests for syphilis were included, unless they were attending exclusively for the monitoring of known chronic HBV infection. Anonymised serum samples were tested for anti-HBc by a passive haemagglutination assay (Green Cross Corporation), with reactive samples being confirmed by a competitive enzyme linked immunosorbent assay (ELISA; Wellcozyme, Wellcome Diagnostics Ltd.). Anti-HIV-1 was detected by gelatin particle agglutination (Serodio-HIV, Fujirebio Inc.) and the results confirmed by competitive ELISA (Wellcozyme). Prior to anonymisation, data was extracted from clinic notes to provide the following : sex, sexual orientation, age, nationality, presenting diagnosis, lifetime number and type of past sexually transmitted diseases (STDs; counting only one episode of genital warts and herpes simplex).

Results were obtained from 1061 of 1074 (98.8%) eligible patients. Bisexual males have been included with homosexual males in all analyses. The number of subjects, their mean age and lifetime number of STDs are shown in Table I.

Table I Demographic and risk factor characteristics

	Males		Females
	Homosexual	Heterosexual	
Number	281	374	406
Mean age (SD)	33.1 (9.09)	30.3 (9.15)	27.1 (7.49)
Mean lifetime no. of STDs (SD)	3.37 (4.08)	1.15 (1.96)	1.1 (2.11)

A univariate analysis of risk factors for anti-HBc seroprevalence was conducted using the SAS software package.

All variables, except age, were dichotomous and for these the Odds ratios were calculated according to the standard method. In the case of age, the estimated parameter is the maximum likelihood estimate (MLE) in a logistic regression model (each one year increase in age multiplies the Odds ratio by the calculated MLE). The numbers in the risk groups were too small to permit a multivariate analysis of risk factors.

Results

The percent seroprevalence of anti-HBc by sexual orientation category is shown in Table II, with 95% confidence intervals.

Table II Seroprevalence of anti-HBc

	Males		Females
	Homosexual	Heterosexual	
%	48.0	7.5	10.8
95% CI	42.2, 53.9	4.8, 10.2	7.8, 13.9

A univariate analysis of risk factors for HBV infection for all patients together shows that all the factors analysed are significantly associated (Table III).

Table III Risk factors for HBV infection (all patients)

Risk factor		Odds ratio	95% CI	p value
Sexual orientation : Heterosexual male vs. homosexual male		0.09	0.05, 0.13	<0.0001
Female vs. homosexual male		0.12	0.08, 0.18	<0.0001
Age in years		1.06*	1.05, 1.08	<0.001
Nationality**	B vs. A	1.67	1.10, 2.55	<0.02
	C vs. A	2.41	1.42, 4.09	<0.001
Lifetime no. STD ≥2 vs. 0 or 1		4.9	3.52, 6.73	<0.0001
Presenting diagnosis STD vs. no STD		0.58	0.41, 0.83	<0.003
HIV-Ab : positive vs. negative		20.6	12.44, 34.12	<0.0001

* Maximum likelihood estimate - see text.
** Nationality categories : A, United Kingdom; B, Europe, Australasia, North America; C, Africa, Indian subcontinent, Middle and Far East, Caribbean, Central and South America.

For homosexuals alone, anti-HBc-seropositivity was significantly associated with increasing age, lifetime number of STDs and HIV-seropositivity (Table IV). European (non-U.K.), Australasian and North American nationality was associated with a 3-fold higher risk of HBV infection compared with UK nationality.

Table IV Risk factors for HBV infection (homosexual males)

Risk factor		Odds ratio	95% CI	p value
Age in years		1.07*	1.04, 1.10	<0.0001
Nationality**	B vs. A	3.08	1.36, 6.97	<0.007
	C vs. A	1.68	0.57, 4.99	N.S.
Lifetime no. STD ≥2 vs. 0 or 1		3.27	1.98, 5.39	<0.0001
Presenting Diagnosis STD vs. no STD		0.61	0.34, 1.07	N.S.
HIV-Ab : positive vs. negative		7.10	3.94, 12.79	<0.0001

* MLE - see text.
** Nationality categories as for Table III.

Amongst heterosexual males, the same risk factors were significantly associated with HBV infection, except that there was only a trend towards an increasing prevalence with increasing age, and the nationality group associated with an increased risk differed (Table V).

Table V Risk factors for HBV infection (heterosexual males)

Risk factor		Odds ratio	95% CI	p value
Age in years		1.04*	1.0, 1.07	N.S. (p=0.06)
Nationality**	B vs A	2.44	0.84, 7.10	N.S.
	C vs A	6.36	2.34, 17.3	<0.0003
Lifetime no. STD ≥2 vs. 0 or 1		2.36	1.05, 5.3	0.037
Presenting Diagnosis STD vs. no STD		1.11	0.50, 2.44	N.S.
HIV-Ab : positive vs. negative		43.1	4.32, 43.04	0.0013

* MLE - see text.
** Nationality categories as for Table III.

Anti-HBc-seropositivity among female patients was not associated with HIV-seropositivity, or number of STDs or the presenting diagnosis of an STD. The only significant associations were with age and nationality (Table VI).

Table VI Risk factors for HBV infection (females)

Risk factor		Odds ratio	95% CI	p value
Age in years		1.05*	1.01, 1.09	<0.02
Nationality**	B vs. A	1.74	0.74, 4.07	N.S.
	C vs. A	4.78	1.91, 12.0	<0.0009
Lifetime no. STD ≥2 vs. 0 or 1		1.66	0.69, 4.0	N.S.
Presenting diagnosis STD vs. no STD		0.73	0.34, 1.59	N.S.
HIV-Ab : positive vs. negative		3.07	0.31, 30.2	N.S.

* MLE - see text.
** Nationality categories as for Table III.

Discussion

We have determined the prevalence of anti-HBc as a marker of past or current HBV infection in a population attending an GUM clinic. The prevalence amongst homosexual or bisexual males is the same as that obtained in an earlier study, (13) and similar to other GUM clinic studies referred to above. The prevalence amongst heterosexuals, both male and female is also higher than the 0.5-1% found in comparable blood donor populations (DR Howell, personal communication), compatible with heterosexual activity being a risk factor for HBV infection. This is supported by the association, in the case of heterosexual males, between anti-HBc prevalence and a history of at least 2 previous STDs, HIV-seropositivity, and a trend towards an association with increasing age. Among female patients, there was a trend towards an association with number of past STDs but this was not significant. For both heterosexual males and females there was also a strong association with origin (nationality) from regions with a higher general population prevalence of HBV infection. The numbers in this study were insufficient to allow a multivariate analysis of these factors.

In the analysis of all groups combined (Table III) there was a significant association between anti-HBc-seropositivity and the absence of an STD diagnosed at that visit to the clinic. This may be attributable to the practice of attendance for routine check-ups by some patients, including particularly those at higher risk of acquiring STDs. The association was not strong enough to be significant in the analysis of any one sexual orientation group alone.

Data on injecting drug use was not collected systematically so that it was not possible to identify all those patients with this as a risk factor for HBV infection, although a later study has suggested that only approximately 2% of patients attending the same clinic in 1990 admitted to ever injecting drugs (manuscript in preparation). A further possible risk factor for HBV infection is number of different sexual partners. Data on partner number was not recorded in this study, however this has been included in the later study refered to above.

This study indicates that both heterosexuals and homosexuals attending an GUM clinic in London are at increased risk of having HBV infection. Individuals of non-U.K. origin are particularly at risk, and there is a variable association with a history of previous STDs. Further studies are being conducted to identify more clearly the characteristics of subgroups within GUM clinic attenders with higher prevalences of HBV infection.

Acknowledgements

Dr Gilson is supported by the Clinical Research and Development Committee of the University College and Middlesex School of Medicine. We thank Dr R.S. Tedder for helpful discussions, and Mr Peter Williams for statistical assistance.

References

1. Fulford KWM, Dane DS, Catterall RD, et al. (1973) Lancet ii: 1470.
2. Coleman JC, Waugh M, Dayton R. (1977) Br J Vener Dis 53: 132.
3. Ellis WR, Murray-Lyon IM, Coleman JC et al. (1979) Lancet ii: 903.
4. Hentzer B, Skinhoj P, Hoybye G, Nielsen AO, Kvorning SA, Faber V. (1980) Scand J Infect Dis 12: 245.
5. Schreeder MT, Thompson SE, Hadler SC et al. (1982) J Infect Dis 146: 7.
6. Christopher PJ, Mailer PT, Crewe EB, Murphy AM. (1984) Aust NZ J Med 14: 491.
7. Hess G, Bienzle U, Slusarczyk J, Hansson BG, Büschenfelde KHM. (1986) Liver 6: 13.
8. Mele A, Franco E, Caprilli F, et al. (1988) Eur J Epidemiol 4: 488.
9. Centers for Disease Control. (1988) MMWR 37: 429, 437.
10. Alter MJ, Coleman PJ, Alexander WJ, et al. (1989) JAMA 262: 1201.
11. Polakoff S. (1990) J Infect 20: 163.
12. Loveday C, Pomeroy L, Weller IVD, et al. (1989) Br Med J 298: 419.
13. Carne CA, Weller IVD, Johnson AM et al. (1987) Lancet ii: 656.

© 1990 Elsevier Science Publishers B.V. (Biomedical Division)
Hepatitis B: A sexually transmitted disease in heterosexuals.
P. Piot and F.E. Andre, editors

Epidemiologic study of the seroprevalence of hepatitis B in patients with sexually transmitted diseases

L. OLMOS*, J.L. VILATA*, A. RODRIGUEZ PICHARDO*

*STD Centres of Madrid, Valencia and Seville.

Introduction

Hepatitis B has traditionally been regarded as a disease which is transmitted by the parenteral or post-transfusional route. However, starting in the seventies, sexual transmission has achieved wide recognition as one of the main transmission routes of this disease in Western countries (1-5).

In a study carried out by the Centers for Disease Control in the U.S.A., a history of multiple sexual partners over the last six months was found to be more frequent among patients with acute hepatitis B than among a control group from the general population (6). Heterosexual activity with multiple partners as the sole risk factor was the probable source of infection in 14% of the cases of hepatitis B. In addition, 9% of the patients developed the infection through heterosexual contacts with HBsAg positive subjects (6). The conclusions of an epidemiologic study conducted in Sweden indicated that the sexual route of transmission was the most frequent route of transmission of hepatitis B (7).

The aim of this study was to determine the seroprevalence of hepatitis B in patients in which sexually transmitted disease (STD) is the sole risk factor and to discover whether this prevalence is related to heterosexual activity with multiple partners and the number of episodes of STD, when it is considered separately from other risk factors.

Material and methods

The sample studied consisted of 624 patients who came to hospital seeking treatment for episodes of sexually transmitted diseases. The patients were seen in the outpatient STD consulting room of three hospitals. These were the Clinical Hospital of Madrid, Clinical Hospital of Seville and General Hospital of Valencia. The recruitment period extended from October 1989 to February 1990. A questionnaire specifically designed for this study was filled out for the patients who came to the STD consultation room over this period. The data gathered referred to personal demographic factors: age, sex, race, education, and place of residence (this last factor led to a division of patients into two groups: those residing in the provincial capital and those residing elsewhere within the same province) and risk factors for STD (number of sexual partners over the last six months, number of episodes of STD throughout the patient's lifetime and diagnosis of present disease). Data was also collected in order to exclude patients having other known risk factors for hepatitis B, apart from sexually transmitted disease. Based on this, homosexuals, intravenous drug addicts, prostitutes, persons who had been in contact with blood or other body fluids, health care personnel and persons with a known history of hepatitis B, were excluded. Blood samples were taken from the patients included in the study for HBsAg, anti-HBs, anti-HBc determinations. The analysis of these markers was performed using the ELISA method (Organon Hepagnostica).

Statistical analysis was carried out by Student's t test when quantitative variables were compared and by Chi^2 test in the case of qualitative variables (Fisher's test was used in pertinent cases).

Results

Of the 624 patients who were initially included in the study, 183 were excluded due to the presence of one of the known risk factors. Thus, the study included 441 heterosexual patients with sexually transmitted diseases. These were distributed geographically as follows: 169 in Madrid, 165 in Valencia, and 107 in Seville.

The distribution of the sample by sex was 290 men (65.7%) and 151 women (34.3%). The mean age was 31.5 years and ages ranged from 17-73 years.

Table I shows the data referring to age, sex, place of residence, number of sexual partners over the last six months, and number of episodes of STD for the three populations. The three populations were only statistically different ($p < 0.01$) with respect to the place of residence. Statistical differences were found when the proportion of subjects residing in the capital was compared to those residing in other places within the province.

Table I Description of the study population

	Madrid	(n=169)	Valencia	(n=165)	Seville	(n=107)
	mean	range	mean	range	mean	range
Age (years)	33.5	18-70	31.1	18-59	29.8	17-56
No. of partners over the last 6 months	3.1	0-21	2.2	2.24	3	1-35
No. of episodes STD	1.4	1-4	1.7	1-15	2	1-12
Sex (%)						
Male/Female	59.7/40.2		67.2/32.2		72.8/27.1	
Residence*						
Provincial capital /other locations	137 /32		97/68		76/31	

* $p < 0.01$; $Chi^2 = 19.6$.

Table II shows the results obtained for hepatitis B prevalence, considered as positive results for any of the three markers tested, and the percentage of carriers (HBsAg positive subjects). It can be seen that there was no difference in prevalence between Madrid and Seville, although differences were noted between either of these and Valencia.

Table II Hepatits B prevalence and chronic carriers

	Total	Madrid	Valencia	Seville
n	441	169	165	107
Any positive marker	84 (19.9%)	38 (22.5%)	20 (12.1%)*	26 (24.3%)
HBsAg	10 (2.2%)	5 (2.9%)	1 (0.6%)*	4 (3.7%)

*p<0.05 Valencia vs. Madrid and Seville.

Table III lists the percentages of positive results for the markers assessed (HBsAg, Anti-HBs and Anti-HBc) for the overall sample. The overall prevalence of hepatitis B virus markers was 19.9%, with a 2.3% prevalence of carriers.

Table III Percentage of positive markers (HBs Ag, anti-HBs and anti-HBc) obtained

	No. of positives (n=441)	%
HBs Ag	10	2.3 %
Anti-HBs	17	4.3 %
Anti-HBc	18	4.3 %
Anti-HBs and Anti HBc	39	9.1 %
Total	84	19.9 %

Table IV compares the prevalence obtained in the three populations for subjects residing in the capital versus those residing outside the capital city. No statistical differences were found in any of the populations for patients residing within the same province.

The results for hepatitis B prevalence according to the patients' sexually transmitted diseases are shown in Table V.

Table IV Prevalence in the study population according to residence in the capital or elsewhere within the same province

	Madrid (n=169)	Valencia (n=165)	Seville (n=07)
Capital	28/137 (20.4%)	11/97 (11.3%)	18/76 (23.6%)
Other locations	10/ 32 (31.2%)	9/68 (13.2%)	8/31 (25.8%)

The results obtained with respect to the variables "number of STD episodes" and "number of sexual partners over the last six months" are listed in Table VI. No statistically significant differences were found on comparing the group of patients with one episode throughout his/her lifetime with those who had two or more. Similarly, no differences were found betweeen those individuals with one sexual partner over the last six months and those who had two or more partners.

Table V Diagnosis of STD and prevalence in the study sample

Diagnosis	Any HBV marker
Chancroid	1/4 (25%)
Herpes	2/8 (25%)
Condylomas	29/121 (23.96%)
Candidas	13/58 (22.4%)
Trichomonas	3/14 (21.4%)
Syphilis	7/42 (16.6%)
Non-gonococcic urethritis	12/75 (16%)
Balanitis	3/21 (14.2%)
Gonococcal infections	7/73 (13.6%)
Chlamydia	0/8 (0%)
Other STD	4/17(23.5%)

Table VI Relation to prevalence with no. STD episodes in lifetime and no. of partners in previous 6 months

No. of STD episodes	Any positive marker (%)
1	42/259 (16.2)
2-3	24/136 (17.6)
4	3/13 (23.07)
No. partners over the last 6 months	**Any positive marker (%)**
0-1	31/214 (14.6)
2-3	20/112 (17.8)
4	18/98 (18.3)

Table VII Distribution of prevalence and chronic carriers by sex

	Any positive marker (%)	HBs Ag positive (%)
Male	61/290 (21.0%)	7/290 (2.4%)
Female	23/151 (15.2%)	3/151 (2.0%)

With respect to the distribution of prevalence by sex (Table VII), no statistically significant differences were noted in prevalence rates between the sexes nor in the number of chronic carriers.

Discussion

Hepatitis B is a disease transmitted by the parenteral or sexual route (horizontal transmission) (6, 8) or by an infected mother to her newborn offspring (vertical transmission) (10,11). The percentage of carriers worldwide ranges from 0.1 to 0.2% in the U.K., the U.S.A., and Scandinavia, to more than 3% in Greece and Southern Italy, and reaches 10-15% in Africa and the Far East (8).

In Spain, the percentage of carriers ranges around 1.4% (11), with a global prevalence of positive markers in the general population of about 18% (12).

In studies carried out in Spain in the groups previously described as being at risk, prevalence rates varying from 18.4-27.4% were found in health care personnel (13, 14), and up to 83.68% in drug addicts (15). In a study carried out in Spain in 1986 on the prevalence of hepatitis B in STD patients, prevalence was found to be 45%, with a 3% rate of HBsAg positive subjects (16). It should be noted, however, that the latter study was carrried out on soldiers during their military service in Madrid (15). In addition, the authors considered that "another possible bias could result from the circumstance that all the sexually transmitted disease patients included in the sample could have been infected by professional prostitutes of a specific zone of the capital city Madrid who may have high HBV infection rates" (16). Therefore, these results cannot be used for comparison with ours.

The results obtained in our study for the overall sample with respect to prevalence (19.9%) and chronic carriers (2.2%) indicate that in the population studied hepatitis B could be considered to have medium endemicity (17).

In the population studied in Madrid and Seville prevalence was 22.5% and 24.3%, respectively (2.9% and 3.7% of HBsAg positive subjects), while in Valencia the percentages were 12.1% and 0.6%, respectively. Based on these results we can conclude that the populations of STD patients studied in Madrid and Seville fall within those considered of medium endemicity (between 2-7% of carriers in the population) (17), and that this prevalence is comparable to that found in other groups considered to be at risk, such as health care personnel. In studies carried out in the latter risk group, a prevalence of 22.5% and 21.2% was found in hospitals of Madrid (18) and Seville (19), respectively.

As for Valencia, the results obtained seem to indicate a prevalence comparable to that of a normal population in areas of low endemicity (17). This data does not accord with expected results for this type of patients nor with the results obtained in this study for Madrid and Seville. It is difficult to attribute the cause of this discrepancy to one specific factor due to the design of the present study: it was an observational study based on a large group of subjects studied at a specific point in time. Analysis of the three study populations revealed that they only differ statistically with respect to the place of residence; the Valencia sample showed a higher proportion of subjects residing outside the capital versus those residing in the capital city than was found in either Madrid or Seville.

Nevertheless, no statistically significant differences were found between the populations residing in the capital and those residing outside it, in any one of the three populations studied. Therefore, the results obtained for Valencia cannot be attributed to this factor.

With relation to the parameter used to evaluate sexual promiscuity (number of sexual partners over the last six months), it can be seen that there were no differences between individuals with one partner and those who had two or more.

On analysis of the results according to the specific STD involved, we observed that there was no type of STD which stood out as a having higher prevalence of HBV infection than the rest. These results contradict those of other studies (16, 20-23) in which a significant correlation was found between syphilis and prevalence of hepatitis B.

The conclusion which may be drawn from our results are that the STD patient populations of Madrid and Seville fall within those considered to be of medium endemicity for hepatitis B, with a higher prevalence in the study sample of these two populations than in the general population (23.2% versus 18%) (12). More remarkably, the percentage of carriers in these populations was 133% higher than the accepted prevalence recognized in Spain (3.3% versus 1.4% (11)). This led us to consider, as other authors have shown, that the presence of STD can be associated with a hepatitis B prevalence rate higher than that found in the general population (4, 24). On the other hand, it should be pointed out that contrary to what has been observed in this type of patient by other authors (4, 6, 24), sexual promiscuity within the STD population seems to have a lower specific weight on the prevalence of hepatitis B. This led us to conclude that in this population the presence of a STD is a more important risk factor than sexual promiscuity.

References

1. Hersh T, Melnick LJ, Goyal RK et al (1971) N Engl J Med 285: 1363.
2. Wright RA (1975) JAMA 232: 717.
3. Redeker AG, Mosley JW, Gocke DJ et al (1975) N Engl J Med 293: 1055.
4. Szmuness W, Much MI, Prince AM et al (1975) Ann Intern Med 83: 489.
5. Heathcote J and Sherlock S (1973) Lancet 1: 1468.
6. Alter MJ, Coleman PJ, Alexander WJ, et al (1989) JAMA 262 (9): 1201.
7. Struve J, Giesecke J, Gudrun L et al (1990) J Infect 20: 111.
8. Sherlock S (1990) Vaccine 8 (suppl 1): S6.
9. Esteban J, Esteban R, Seijo G et al (1984) An Med Int (Madr) 4: 112.
10. Derso A, Boxall E, Tarlow MJ, et al (1978) Br Med J 1: 949.
11. Genesca J, Esteban JI, Esteban R et al (1986) Med Clin 87: 271.
12. Vargas V, Pedreira JD, Esteban R et al (1982) Med Clin 78: 265.
13. Villate JI, Aguirre C, Corral JM, et al (1985) Med Clin 84: 85.
14. Garcîa Bengoechea M, Cortês A, Francisco C, Cosme A, Arriola A, et al (1987) Med Clin (Barc) 88: 179.

15. Santamarîa Jauregui JM, Sadaba Garay CF, Martînez Odriogola P, et al (1984) Med Clin (Barc) 82: 13.
16. Requena Caballero L, Vazquez Lôpez F, Arjona Manuel C, et al (1986) Med Clin (Barc) 87: 309.
17. Center for Disease Control (1990) MMWR 39: No. RR-2: 5.
18. Juanes JR, Fuertes A, Lagos E, et al (1987) Rev Esp Microbial Clîn (2) 4: 225.
19. Sanchez-Guijarro, Rivera F, Lissen E, Ollero M, et al (1984) Med Clîn (Barc) 83: 1.
20. Brugera M, Sanchez-Tapias J M, Latorre X, et al (1984) Med Clin (Barc) 83: 869.
21. Kryger P, Petersen NS, Mathiesen L, et al (1982) J Infect Dis 145: 23.
22. Bleeker A, Coutinho RA, Bakker-Kok J, et al (1981) Br J Vener Dis 57: 196.
23. Baker-Zander SA, Sell S, Lukerhart SA (1982) Infect Immun 37: 568.
24. Alter MJ, Ahtone J, Weisfuse I, et al (1986) JAMA 256(10): 1307.

Heterosexual transmission of hepatitis B in Amsterdam

CHRISTA HOOYKAAS, ROEL A. COUTINHO, GERARD J.J. VAN DOORNUM

Municipal Health Service, Department of Public Health, Nieuwe Achtergracht 100, 1018 WT Amsterdam, The Netherlands

Introduction

Sexual transmission of hepatitis B virus (HBV) , among other modes of transmission, has received more attention in the last decade. Several studies have indicated that the risk for HBV infection increases with the multiplicity of sexual partners, as well as with a history of multiple episodes of Sexually Transmitted Diseases (STDs) (1-5). We did a study among heterosexual men and women with multiple partners to assess the risk factors for heterosexual transmission of HBV.

Material and methods

Study group

Heterosexual men and women with 5 or more different sexual partners in the preceding 6 months, were recruited from visitors of a STD-clinic of the Municipal Health Service of Amsterdam, The Netherlands. The study was designed to measure the prevalence and incidence and determine the risk factors of Human Immunodeficiency Virus (HIV) infection among heterosexuals. We therefore excluded haemophiliacs, men with homosexual contacts and intravenous drug users in the preceding 5 years. Participation was on a voluntary basis.

Besides recording their demographic characteristics, participants were extensively interviewed about their sexual lifestyle (e.g. type and number of partners, frequency of different sexual techniques and condom use) history of STDs and they were examined for STDs according to a standard protocol. Blood samples were taken to test for antibodies against HIV, HBV and *Treponema pallidum.*

Serological methods

Testing for HBV-markers was performed using commercial kits: Ausab EIA (Abbott) for antibodies to hepatitis B surface antigen (anti-HBs) and using Corzyme (Abbott) for antibodies to hepatitis B core antigen (anti-HBc). Samples solely reactive for anti-HBc were also tested for hepatitis B surface antigen (HBsAg) using the Auszyme assay (Abbott). All sera were also tested for antibodies to HIV (Abbott Recombinant HTLV-III EIA), and confirmation of reactive or borderline samples was carried out in a Western immunoblot (Biotech/Dupont WIB). Screening for syphilis was carried out using the *Treponema pallidum* hemagglutination assay (TPHA, Furijebo) and reactive sera were retested with the Veneral Disease Research Laboratory (VDRL, Wellcome) test and the Fluorescent *Treponema* Absorption test (FTA-Abs).

Table I General characteristics of 579 heterosexuals from HBV low and middle endemic countries by gender

Characteristic	Low Endemic		Middle Endemic	
	Men n=133	Women n=245	Men n=113	Women n= 88
Mean (sd) age in years	34 (10)	29 (7)	30 (8)	29 (7)
% Living in Amsterdam	78%	77%	95%	80%
% with private partners				
in the preceding 5 years	93%	98%	86%	97%
mean number partners	45	25	52	9
in the preceding 4 months	84%	90%	67%	76%
mean number partners	5.7	3.8	6.4	2.9
% with commercial partners				
in the preceding 5 years	74%	72%	81%	92%
in the preceding 4 months	55%	67%	69%	89%
mean number partners	6.5	87*	9.1	135*
% with high risk partner				
in the preceding 5 years **	29%	39%	34%	22%
% who reported STDs ***				
in the preceding 5 years	38%	45%	55%	33%
in the preceding 4 months	7%	7%	17%	7%
% diagnosed with STDs ****				
at entry of the study	20%	24%	35%	27%

* Mean number of clients per month, in preceding 4 months.
** High risk partners are intravenous drug users, bisexual men and persons from AIDS-endemic regions.
*** Included STDs were: syphilis, gonorrhoea, *Chlamydia trachomatis* infection and genital herpes.
**** Included STDs were: syphilis, gonorrhoea, *Chlamydia trachomatis* infection, newly acquired genital herpes, trichomonas, newly acquired condylomata accuminata and HIV-infections.

Results

Study group

From October 1987 through December 1989, 598 men and women participated; 381 were born in HBV low endemic countries (LEC) - North/Western Europe and North America - 205 were born in HBV middle endemic countries (MEC) - Mediterranean countries, Latin America and Eastern Europe - and 12 originated from HBV high endemic countries (HEC). Participants from HEC, and those participants from LEC and MEC who reported to be vaccinated against HBV (3 from LEC, 4 from MEC) were excluded from further analyses.

The participants had a mean age of 30 years, but men were older than women. Most participants had 1 or more private partners in the preceding 5 years, but men had more partners in the preceding 5 years and the preceding 4 months. More than half the participants had had commercial partners (either prostitutes or clients); men and women from MEC had more commercial partners than participants from LEC. More than 40% reported to have had 1 or more episodes of STDs (Table I).

As serological evidence for prior HBV-infection, we used the criterion of 1 or more positive HBV-markers. The HBV-prevalence for men and women from LEC was respectively 13/133 (10%) and 25/245 (10%), and for men and women from MEC respectively 47/113 (42%) and 17/88 (19%) (Table II). Only 6 HBsAg carriers were found, all men from MEC.

Table II Serology of 579 heterosexuals with multiple partners from HBV low and middle endemic countries by gender

	Low endemic		Middle endemic	
	Men	Women	Men	Women
	n=133	n=245	n=113	n= 88
No. (%) HBV-markers				
anti-HBc- and anti-HBs-	120 (90)	223 (90)	66 (58)	71 (81)
anti-HBc+ and anti-HBs+	10 (8)	15 (6)	31 (27)	14 (16)
anti-HBc+ and anti-HBs-	3 (2)	5 (2)	10 (9)	2 (2)
anti-HBc- and anti-HBs+	0 (0)	5 (2)	6 (5)	1 (1)
No. (%) TPHA positive	3 (2)	7 (3)	9 (8)	5 (6)
No. (%) HIV positive	0 (0)	0 (0)	1 (1)	1 (1)

Altogether, the HBV-prevalence among persons from MEC was 32%, which is significantly higher than the prevalence among persons from LEC (10%) . As the transmission route for most persons from MEC is likely to be different from that of persons from LEC, these two groups were analysed seperately concerning the risk factors for heterosexual transmission.

LEC

HBV-positive men and women had more often sexual contact with a high risk person (intravenous drug users, bisexual men or persons from AIDS-endemic regions) in the preceding 5 years than HBV-negative participants ($p < 0.05$, one-tail). HBV-positive participants also had more often a history of STDs, but this difference was not significant. The only significant risk factor which emerged from a stepwise discriminant analysis (a significant change in Rao's V as criterion) was sexual contact with a high risk partner in the preceding 5 years. A self-reported history of STDs in the preceding 5 years and diagnosed STDs had only a minor influence. (Table IV). No associations were found with the number of private or commercial partners in the preceding 5 years or 4 months, or the number of 'unprotected' vaginal contacts with private or commercial partners.

Table III Risk factors for HBV-positivity in 378 heterosexuals with multiple partners from HBV low endemic countries

Risk factor	Men: HBV-markers		Women: HBV-markers	
	Pos.	Neg.	Pos.	Neg.
	n= 13	n=120	n= 25	n=220
No. (%) who had contact with risk partner (5 years)	7 (54)	32 (27)	15 (60)	80 (36)
No. (%) who reported STDs				
in the preceding 5 years	6 (46)	44 (37)	16 (64)	95 (43)
in the preceding 4 months	2 (15)	7 (6)	2 (8)	15 (7)
No. (%) diagnosed with STDs at entry of the study	4 (31)	23 (19)	8 (32)	50 (23)

Table IV Prediction of HBV-positivity in 378 heterosexuals with multiple partners from HBV low endemic countries (stepwise discriminant analysis)

Risk factor	RAO's V	Significance of change	
1 or more high risk partner	9.5	0.002	
1 or more reported STDs (5 years)	13.0	0.06	(NS)
1 or more diagnosed STDs (at entry)	14.8	0.18	(NS)

MEC

More men than women from MEC had positive HBV-markers ($p < 0.01$) , but none of the variables concerning sexual lifestyle or STDs were associated significantly with HBV-positivity.

Discussion

Our study demonstrates that the HBV-prevalence among heterosexuals depends mainly on the country participants originated from. In middle or high endemic countries HBV can be transmitted through heterosexual contact, but other transmission modes cannot be excluded and may be more important. Among heterosexuals the HBV-transmission risk has been reported to be associated with the number of different sexual partners and a history of STDs (1-5). Contrary to these findings, we found that the risk for HBV-infection in heterosexuals with multiple partners from low endemic countries increases if there is a history of sexual contact with a high risk person, and that a history of STDs had only a minor influence. We found no evidence that the number of partners per se had any influence.

Acknowledgements

The authors wish to thank all participants, and personnel of the Clinic for Sexually Transmitted Diseases of the Municipal Health Service of Amsterdam for their necessary help to conduct this study. This study was financially supported by a grant from the Dutch Foundation for Preventive Medicine (grant no. 28-1529[1,2]).

References

1. Judson FN (1981) Sexually Transmitted Diseases 8(supplement): 336.
2. Alter MJ, Ahtone J, Weisfuse I, Starko K, Vacalis TD et al (1986) JAMA 256: 1307.
3. CDC (1988) MMWR 37: 429.
4. Alter MJ, Coleman PJ, Alexander WJ, Kramer E, Miller JK et al (1989) JAMA 262: 1201.
5. CDC (1989) MMWR 38: 818.

© 1990 Elsevier Science Publishers B.V. (Biomedical Division)
Hepatitis B: A sexually transmitted disease in heterosexuals.
P. Piot and F.E. Andre, editors

Hepatitis B virus and heterosexual transmission in Paris, France: Report on 504 patients attending an STD clinic

P. MOREL, F. MORINET, M. JANIER, F. LASSAU, R. MEOUCHY, Y. PEROL

Hôpital Saint Louis, 75475 Paris, France

Introduction

In low endemicity areas, sexual transmission of hepatitis B has long been considered as being mainly a problem of homosexual men (1-4). However, recent epidemiological studies in the USA have shown heterosexual activity to be a risk factor for acquiring hepatitis B (5,6). This has led to recommendations by the CDC that heterosexuals with multiple sexual partners or who seek treatment for sexually transmitted diseases should be vaccinated against this disease (7).

In epidemiological terms, France is a low endemicity country for hepatitis B, comparable in that respect with the USA. As in the USA, studies have shown that sexually active homosexual men in France are at an increased risk of acquiring hepatitis B (8).

Studies of heterosexual transmission of hepatitis B in France are lacking and we wished to investigate the prevalence of hepatitis B virus serological markers in heterosexual patients attending a sexually transmitted disease (STD) clinic in an inner Paris hospital.

Methods

Patients attending the Hôpital Saint Louis STD clinic were eligible to take part in the study. Patients were told the purpose of the study and their informed consent was obtained in writing.

Each patient was interviewed by a physician using a standard questionnaire. Patients having any known risk factor for hepatitis B, other than heterosexual activity, were not included: patients born in high endemicity areas, having a history of homosexual contacts, IV drug injections, professional exposure to human blood or body fluids, prostitution or who were vaccinated against hepatitis B were excluded.

In addition to these risk factors, the following information was sought by means of the questionnaire: age, sex, ethnic group, marital status, country of birth, education level, clinical signs of hepatitis, household or sexual contact with patients with hepatitis, age of first sexual contact, number of sexual partners (total and in the preceding 6 months), previous STD, history of blood transfusion, use of condoms. Eligible patients were tested for hepatitis B surface antigen (HBsAg), for antibodies to HBsAg (anti-HBs) and antibodies to hepatitis B core antigen (anti-HBc). Auszyme, Ausab and Corzyme immunoassays

(Abbott Diagnostics, Rungis, France) were used. Statistical analysis was carried out using S.A.S. software, Chi-square tests were used for correlations.

Results

Five hundred and four patients, of which 70% (351) were men and 30% (153) were women were included over a period of 2 months (February to April 1990). Ages ranged from 16 to 83 years old (mean SD: 34 years ± 12).

Eighty six percent (431) were white, 12% (61) were black, mainly from the West Indies or North Africa, and 2% (12) were either Asians, Hispanics or half-caste.

The two main areas of birth were Europe (46%) and Maghreb (33%); 8% of our patients were born in the West Indies, 2% in Africa and 16% in other low or intermediate endemicity areas. Fifty four percent (271) of our patients had never been married, 36% (182) were married and 10% (51) were divorced or widowed. Eleven percent (55) had received no school education, 53.5% (270) had between 6 and 12 years of education, and 35.5% (179) had over 12 years of education.

Total number of reported sexual partners ranged from zero to 528, with a mean number of 32.5 (SD 51.5); sexual partners in the preceding six months ranged from zero to 50 (mean ± SD: 2.4 ± 4.25).

The mean age of the first sexual contact was 17.5 (SD 3.0) with extremes ranging from 8 to 32 years.

Sixty six percent of the patients had had at least one episode of STD; extremes ranged from no episode to 50 episodes (mean ± SD: 1.6 ± 3.1).

As shown in Table I, the only major difference between men and women in our population seems to lie in the total number of sexual partners declared by the patients; on average men reported 39 partners and women 14.

Table I Mean parameters (±SD)

	All	Men	Women
n	504	351	153
Age	34.4 (11.6)	36.4 (12.1)	29.7 (8.9)
No. of sex partners in past 6 months	2.4 (4.25)	2.6 (4.1)	1.9 (4.6)
Total no. of sex partners	32.5 (51.5)	39.5 (55.7)	14.0 (31.8)
Age of first sexual contact	17.5 (3)	17.3 (2.8)	18.0 (3.2)
Previous STD episodes	1.6 (3.1)	1.8 (3.5)	1.1 (3.1)

Table II shows the prevalence of hepatitis B serological markers in our population sample. One hundred and three men (29.4%) had at least one marker versus 26 (17%) women ($p = 0.003$).

When compared with other sub-groups of the French population (Table III), it appears that higher rates of infection have been previously reported only in male homosexuals or IV drug users (8-14).

Comparison may not be valid because of high percentage of STD patients from endemic areas as compared to other groups.

Table II Prevalence of hepatitis B serological markers

	Total	Men	Women
n	504	351	153
HBsAg %	4.2	5.1	2.0
Anti-HBs %	18.45	20.8	13.1
Anti-HBc %	23.5	26.9	15.7
At least one marker %	25.65	29.4	17.0

Table III Hepatitis B markers in French population sub-groups

	Blood donors	Male military blood donors	Health care personnel	I.V. drug users	Homosexual men
HBsAg%	0.365	0.16	0.34	15	5.5
Anti HBs%	ND	1.1	ND	67**	71.3
Anti HBc%	3.6*	1.7	12		ND
Reference	9	10	12	13	8

*Estimated.
**Anti HBs + Anti HBc.
ND, not determined.

Table IV shows the prevalence rates by age; overall, patients over 36 years of age had a significantly higher incidence of markers: 23% before and 37% after 36 years ($p < 0.001$).

Table IV Percentage of markers according to age

Age(years)	<20	20-25	26-30	31-35	36-40	41-45
n	30	90	111	86	58	47
% markers	16.6	14.4	25.2	16.3	39.7	29.8
Age	46-50	51-55	56-60	61-65	>65	
n	29	19	15	9	9	
% markers	34.5	47.4	33.3	66.7	22.2	

A strong correlation was shown in men between prevalence rate and country of birth: 13.3% of men born in France had at least one marker versus 40.3% in men born in Maghreb countries ($p < 0.001$). The female sub-group was too small to show a similar correlation.

There also exists in both sexes a close correlation between prevalence rate and level of education: the higher the level of education, the lower the prevalence rate (e.g. 48.1% in persons who never went to school and 12.6% in patients with over 12 years of education, ($p < 0.001$)).

Regarding previous STD episodes, a relationship was found (in men only) between the presence of markers and a past episode of syphilis, gonorrhea or condyloma acuminatum ($p = 0.002$); this correlation was not found with other STDs (chlamydia, genital herpes or *Trichomonas vaginalis*).

Higher prevalence rates were found in persons having had 5 or more sexual partners in the preceding 6 months: 57% versus 25% in persons with less than 5 partners ($p = 0.02$). No correlation was found with the total number of sexual partners.

There was no clear relationship between marital status, race, use of condoms, history of blood transfusion, contacts with patients with hepatitis and the presence of serological markers.

Discussion

In this study we found that the main factors which correlated with the presence of serological markers of hepatitis B were: sex (men are more at risk than women, possibly because of their higher number of sexual partners), country of birth (patients from intermediate endemicity areas are more at risk than those from low endemicity areas), age (risk increases two-fold after 36 years of age), history of one or more 'high risk' STD (syphilis, gonorrhea, condyloma), number of partners in the previous 6 months and education level. It is however possible that this last factor reflects, at least partly the relationship between hepatitis B acquisition and birth in an intermediate endemicity area where education is less easily available.

The relationship which was found in men between the presence of markers and a history of syphilis, gonorrhea and/or condyloma, but not with a history of chlamydia, herpes or *Trichomonas vaginalis* may suggest that some STDs are indicators of more 'risky' sexual behaviours than others.

One could be tempted to ascribe the high prevalence rate of serological markers that were found in this study to the high proportion of patients which were born in intermediate endemicity areas for this disease, particularly in Maghreb counties (33% of our patients were born in either Morocco, Algeria or Tunisia).

However, we feel that this fact does not invalidate our findings for two reasons: firstly this 33% figure is not a peculiarity of our clinic but simply reflects the origins of a large part of patients who attend inner city hospitals in France. Secondly, prevalence figures found in patients who were born in France, even though lower than in North African patients, are still much higher than that of the general population (14% rate for all markers and 2.4% for HBsAg) and thus clearly show that heterosexual activity is, in this group of patients, a risk factor for the acquisition of hepatitis B. This 2.4% chronic carrier rate is above the WHO threshold defining population groups in which immunization programmes must be considered.

Conclusion

This study has shown that high prevalence rates of markers of hepatitis B can be found in heterosexual patients who attend STD clinics in Paris.

We thus confirm, as is now accepted in other developed countries, particularly the USA, that hepatitis B is a sexually transmitted disease which affects not only male homosexuals but also sexually active heterosexuals.

Given the high morbidity and mortality related to hepatitis B worldwide, we feel that the CDC and WHO recommendations regarding hepatitis B immunisation should be applied to heterosexuals seeking treatment for STD in France.

We gratefully acknowledge Abbott Diagnostics France's help for providing part of the immunoassay kits, as well as Drs Couroucé and Boulesteix for communicating data on hepatitis B markers in civilian and military blood donors.

References

1. Fulkford KWM, Dane DS (1973) Lancet 1: 1470.
2. Szmuness W, Much MI, Prince AM, Hoofnagle JH, Cherubin CE, Harley EJ, Block GH (1975) Ann Intern Med 83: 489.
3. Dietzman DE, Harnisch JP, Ray CG, Alexander ER. Holmes KK (1977) JAMA 238: 2625.
4. Schreeder MT, Thompson SE, Hadler SC, Berquist KR, Zaidi A, Maynard JE, Ostrow D, Judson FN, Braff EH, Nylund T, Moore JN Jr, Gardner P, Doto IL, Reynolds G (1982) J Infect Dis 146: 5.
5. Alter MJ, Ahtone J, Weisfuse I, Starko K, Demetri Vacalis T, Maynard JE (1986) JAMA 256: 1307.
6. Alter MJ, Coleman PJ, James Alexander W, Kramer E, Miller JK, Mandel E, Hadler SC, Margolis HS (1989) JAMA 262: 1201.
7. Anon. (1990) Morb Mortal Wkly Rep 39 S-2: 1.
8. Ravily V (1985) Thése pour le doctorat en médecine, Université René Descartes, Paris.
9. Couroucé AM (personal communication).
10. Boulesteix G, Bourin P, Fabre G, Blanchard de Vaucouleurs A, Molinié C, Denee JM, Buisson Y, Schill H, Joussemet M (1990) Rev Fr Transfus Hémobiol 33: 9.
11. Roudot-Thoraval F, Kouadja F, Wirquin W, Thiers V, Avons P, Brechot C, Dhumeaux D (1989) Gastroenterol Clin Biol 13: 353.
12. Czernichow P, Caillard JF, Prudent P, Bastard C, Proust B (1985) Rev Epidem et Santé Publ 33: 292.
13. Espinoza P, Bouchard I, Buffet C, Thiers V, Pillot J, Etienne JP (1987) Gastroenterol Clin Biol 11: 288.

© 1990 Elsevier Science Publishers B.V. (Biomedical Division)
Hepatitis B: A sexually transmitted disease in heterosexuals.
P. Piot and F.E. Andre, editors

Heterosexual transmission of hepatitis B in Sweden

MARGARETA BÖTTIGER, BRITH CHRISTENSON

Epidemiological Department, National Bacteriological Laboratory, Stockholm, Sweden

Epidemiological background

Hepatitis B (HB) is included among the communicable diseases that it is mandatory to report in Sweden. The national figures of clinical hepatitis of all types are given in Figure 1. HBsAg carriers are also recorded through laboratory reports. Hepatitis B virus (HBV) of the *ad* type was prevailing at a probably low level before the 1960's when the *ay* type was introduced and spread among intravenous drug users (IVDU). The transmission of HBV to hospital personnel then became a major problem. Since rigid preventive measures were introduced in hospitals in the 1970's this route of transmission was successfully reduced and the incidence among hospital personnel is now equal to that of the whole population. Throughout the last 2 decades intravenous drug users constituted a considerable proportion of the notified cases i.e. around 30% of 480 cases in 1979 and 40-50% of 265 in 1989. In Sweden, as well as in other Scandinavian countries, a decline of clinical hepatitis B was observed after 1985 and was assumed to be related to the preventive measures against the spread of HIV. However, the downward trend of HB was broken in 1989 when both the number of IVDU and sexually infected persons increased. The non-IVDU and sexual transmission category, i.e. persons infected through contact with young adopted children, by blood transfusions and tattooing as well as hospital personnel, amounted to only 10 cases in 1989. Persons sexually infected, persons notified to be 'infected abroad' and infection of unknown origin constituted half of the cases.

The heterosexual cases

The epidemiological information on the different routes of infection improved during the last decade. Well known routes were probably fairly well reported also earlier but 10 years ago we obtained no information regarding mode of infection on almost half of the cases. In the last two years, 1988 and 1989, only 15% belonged to this 'unknown' category. An active effort to obtain more information may have contributed to these results. A recent study carried out in the main hospital for infectious diseases in Stockholm (1) indicated that almost all cases earlier reported as of 'unknown' origin in fact were transmitted by the sexual route.

Not only cases reported as heterosexually transmitted, but also those 'contracted abroad' and those with 'no information obtained' are thus in this presentation regarded as mainly sexually infected. A survey of the notification during the last 10 years where the cases were divided into non-sexual transmission and probable sexual transmission is given in Figure 2.

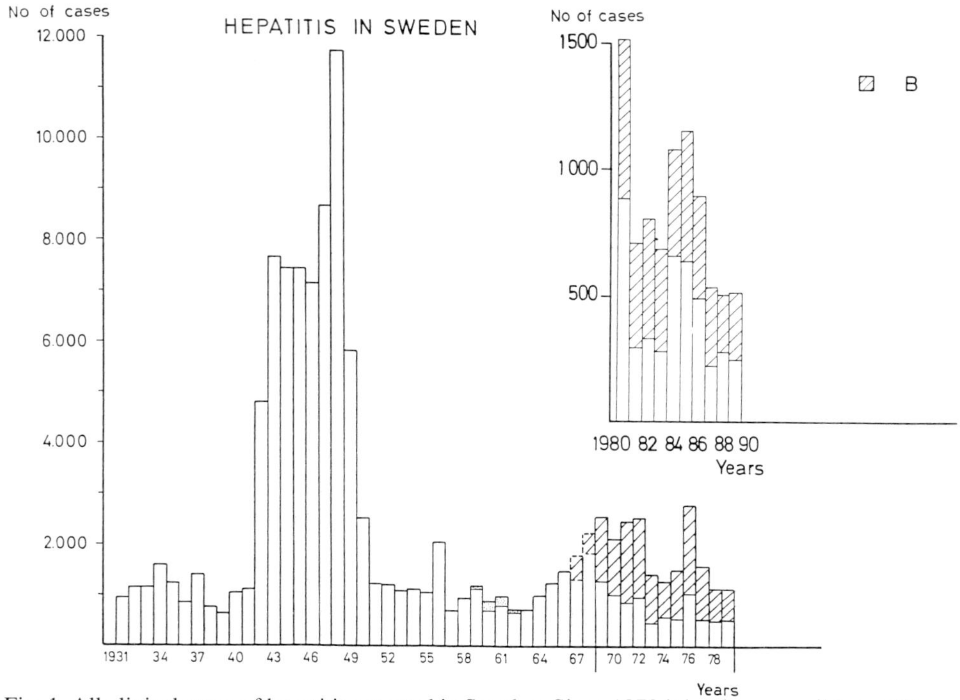

Fig. 1. All clinical cases of hepatitis reported in Sweden. Since 1970 it has been possible to differentiate between hepatitis A and B.

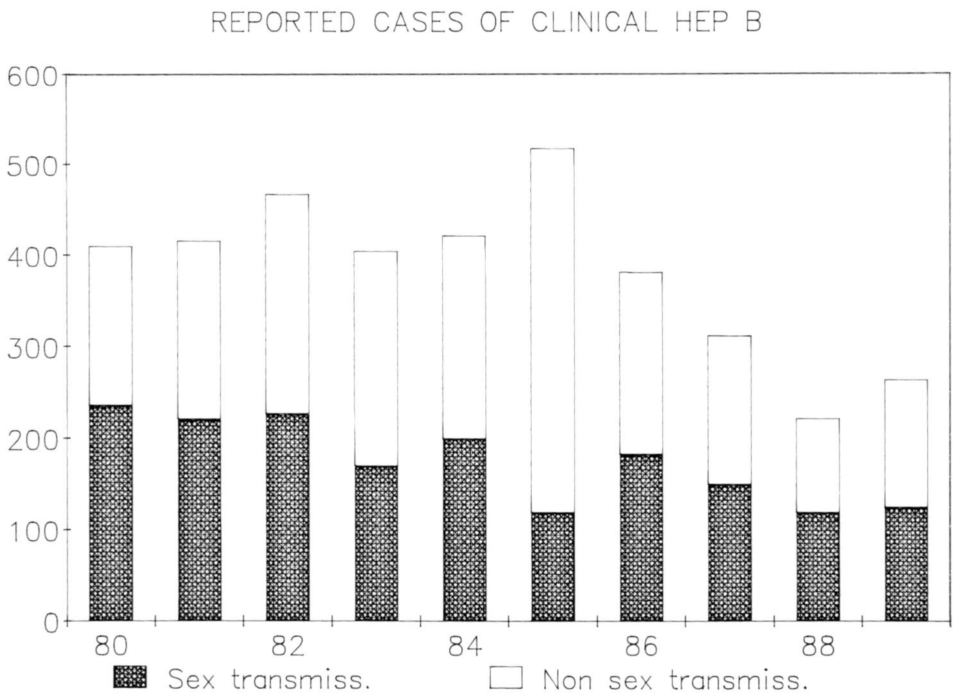

Fig. 2. Hepatitis B cases divided into two categories: i.e. probable sexual transmission and non-sexual transmission.

Table I Heterosexual transmission in patients studied at Roslagstulls Hospital, Stockholm (1985)

Characteristics of partner	No. of patients
IVDU	11
Bisexual men	3
From high endemicity area	11
Recent patient	7
Chronic carrier	10

* One or several characteristics.
From Struve J et al. Journal of Infection 1990; 20:111.

Of the known heterosexually infected persons notified in 1988 and 1989 almost half had information about connection with foreigners and 10% with drug users.

From the detailed study carried out in 1985 at Roslagstulls Hospital in Stockholm (1) the following summary can be given. 78 cases were treated that year and for 66 of them the route of infection could be defined. In total 33 were estimated to be heterosexually infected. In Table I risk factors of the partners are given. Countries mentioned in the patients' histories as place of contact outside Sweden were Mediterranean countries of Europe as well as Portugal, Lebanon, India, Pakistan, Barbados and Brazil. Six patients either came from these or had a family member from these countries.

Carriers of HBV should since July 1989 be notified by physicians. This notification is so far less complete. However, reports have also been sent - directly from the laboratories - for the last 10 years. During the 10 last years the number reported doubled from about 1000 to about 2000. More than 95% are immigrants, mainly refugees from Arabic and African countries.

The HBV carriers among adopted children is another group of concern but are less numerous. About 25-30 patients are reported per year. The majority are HBe antigen carriers. To this can be added at least 50 other verified cases among other young immigrants under 5 years of ages in 1989. We are now beginning to observe secondary cases sexually transmitted from the adopted children when they grow up.

The future scenario is a continued number of Swedes contracting infection, mainly from foreigners, and a considerable importation of HBV carriers. This importation is now at least 2000 per year. The number of potential spreaders is thus increasing at a considerable rate. Among native Swedes without specific risk factors the HBsAg carriership is 0.05-0.1%. In contrast to the Swedes the foreigners are to a much higher degree also HBe-antigen carriers as the majority of them were infected in childhood.

If the influx of refugees from high endemic areas continues we will encounter an increasing number of heterosexual HB transmission also among the now non-immune Swedish population.

Reference

1. Struve J, Giesecke J, Lindh G and Weiland O (1990) J Infect 20, 111.

Hepatitis B: A sexually transmitted disease in heterosexuals.
P. Piot and F.E. Andre, editors

Seroepidemiological study of HBV-markers in STD patients in Austria

ANGELIKA STARY[1], WOLFGANG KOPP[2], CLAUDIA VITOUCH[1]

[1] *Ambulatory for Diagnosis of Infectious Venero-dermatological Diseases, Vienna, Austria and* [2] *Department for STD Control, Public Health Centre, Vienna, Austria*

Introduction

Many studies indicate that both heterosexual and homosexual intercourse may be associated with transmission of the hepatitis B virus (HBV). The high prevalence of hepatitis B among male homosexuals is well documented and HBV markers are recorded in up to 80% of this special risk group (1). One of the main factors for this high prevalence is the highly promiscuous sexual activity of homosexuals. There is also considerable evidence that transmission of HBV can occur by heterosexual contact as well. Sexual partners of individuals with acute hepatitis B are at increased risk of acquiring HBV when compared with other members of the household. The presence of HBV in vaginal secretions, saliva, as well as in semen demonstrates the possible transmission not only by blood but also by heterosexual contact with infectious persons (2).

The prevalence of HBV in heterosexuals varies depending on promiscuous behaviour and the number of other STDs and is higher in prostitutes (3) than in the population at large (4). However, the incidence of HBV markers in different groups of heterosexuals is less well documented in many European countries. In the present study a screening for HBV markers was performed in two groups of heterosexual STD patients in Vienna to establish the prevalence of HBV in different risk groups.

Patients and methods

Patients

The study was performed in a selected group of 497 male and female patients attending two different STD outpatient clinics identified as A and B for the puposes of this study. Based on the information obtained on the history of hepatitis, medically related work, history of intravenous drug abuse as well as sexual activity and number of partners during the last six months, 36 persons were excluded due to a history of known risk factors for transmission of HBV other than heterosexual promiscuous behaviour. Prostitutes were excluded as well.

Methods

Serum samples were obtained from 149 male and 312 female patients in total. Group A consisted of 58 male and 51 female patients and group B 312 females and 149 males; all were tested for HBV. Hepatitis B surface antigen (HBsAg), antibody to HBsAg (anti-HBs) and antibody to hepatitis core antigen (anti-HBc) were determined by using a commercially available enzyme linked immunosorbent test (Auszyme monoclonal™ , Ausab EIA™ , Corzyme™, Abbott Lab., USA). Serologic evidence of HBV infections was defined by any positive result in at least one serologic marker.

Most of the patients were also screened for other STDs such as syphilis, gonorrhea HIV, *Chlamydia trachomatis* and yeast infections (5).

The frequency of HBV markers was compared with the results of other STDs and the behaviour of heterosexual activity as characterised by the number of sexual partners and the number of STDs. This was evaluated by computer assisted methods (chi^2 -test, Mann-Whitney's U-Test).

Results

Hepatitis B

Out of the 461 persons 51 (11.1%) were positive for at least one HBV marker (Table I). Of the 107 patients tested in group A 30 (28.0%) had a positive result (20 males, 10 females), whereas only 21 (5.9%) (5 males, 16 females) of the 354 persons tested in group B had a positive result in at least one HBV marker. In Table I the results in the different HBV markers are listed: in both groups most of the positive patients showed anti-HBc (93.3%, 85.7%). Only 3 persons out of the 51 positive patients were HBsAg positive in addition to a positive result for anti-HBc.

Table I Prevalence of HBV markers in STD patients

Patients	HBV n (% pos.)*	HBsAg n (% pos.)*	anti-HBs n (% pos.)*	anti-HBc n (%pos.)*
Total number n= 461	51 (11.1)	3 (5.9)	38 (74.5)	46 (90.2)
Group A n= 107	30 (28.0)	2 (6.7)	20 (66.7)	28 (93.3)
Group B n= 354	21 (5.9)	1 (4.8)	18 (85.7)	18 (85.7) *

*% of HBV positive patients; (n= 51).

Epidemiological data

Marital status. There was no significant difference between HBV-positive and HBV-negative persons concerning their marital status.

History of hepatitis. A history of hepatitis was remembered by 3.7% (17/454) of all questioned persons (Table II). Among the HBV positives, 18.2% had a history of clinical symptoms of HBV (group A 8.7%, group B 28.6%). A close contact to a HBV-positive person was known by 5.6% of all persons included in this study. Out of the HBV-positive patients of group B 19% remembered a close contact to a HBV-positive person, but none of those of group A.

Table II History of hepatitis B

	All persons Pos and neg.	Group A Positive	Group B Positive
History of clinical symptoms	3.7%	8.7%	28.6%
Close contact with HBV-positive person	5.6%	0.0%	19.0%

Sexual activity. The promiscuous activity of the persons included in the study was based on the information given about the number of sexual partners and the history of genital infections. Heterosexual activity differed significantly in both groups (Table III). Promiscuous activity was reported by about two-thirds of patients belonging to group A compared with only 3.9% of those of group B. 70.9% of patients of group A but only 16.0% of those of group B reported more than one sexual partner.

Table III Sexual behaviour of two groups of STD patients

	GROUP A % (Yes/total)	GROUP B % (Yes/total)
Promiscuous	62.5 (65/104)	3.9 (14/355)
Sexual partners		
2-5	41.7 (10/24)	15.1 (52/344)
>5	29.2 (7/24)	0.9 (3/344)
Genital infections	100.0 (106/106)	86.2 (306/355)
1st time	55.7 (59/106)	47.2 (144/305)
>3 times	19.8 (21/106)	4.9 (15/305)

The promiscuous activity differed not only between both groups, but also between males and females: more than one partner was remembered by 40% of the 144 males and by 10.4% of the 311 females in the last 6 months. 35.4% of the males but only 7.7% of the females gave information about promiscuous activity.

Genital infections. No significant differences were found between patients of both groups in relation to genital infections at the time of sampling, since this was the reason to attend the outpatient clinics and the criteria for inclusion into this study. However, significant differences were found when data were obtained about the history of past genital infections. 19.8% of the patients belonging to group A and only 4.9% of the other group remembered more than three genital infections in the past. So far, the data on the sexual behaviour of persons demonstrate the significant differences between both groups. Group A can therefore be considered as a 'high-risk' STD group in comparison with group B as a 'low-risk' STD group.

HBV and other STDs

Prevalence of other STDs in group A and group B. Most of the patients were screened for STDs such as syphilis, gonorrhea, HIV, *C. trachomatis* and yeast infections according to their clinical symptoms or history of contacts. Serological evidence of syphilis was observed in 38 out of the 201 persons (18.9%), most of them already treated. Gonorrhea was diagnosed in 11.8% and *C. trachomatis* in 10.9% of all cases. Four patients showed antibodies against HIV. Yeast infections were found in 23.7% of all patients included in this study.

Prevalence of HBV and other STDs. The highest prevalence of *HBV* markers was found in patients with serological evidence of syphilis (Table IV) . 42.1% of the syphilis-positive patients were also positive for HBV compared with 16.6% in the syphilis-negative ones ($p = 0.0005$). Of the patients infected with *Neisseria gonorrhoeae* 25.9% revealed a positive result for HBV. Out of the four HIV positive patients one person was also positive for HBV. The lowest coincidence of HBV with other STDs was found in those with genital yeast infections.

Table IV Prevalence of HBV-markers in patients with other STDs

STD	No. positive cases	Prevalence
Syphilis		
n = 38	16	42.1%
Gonorrhea		
n = 54	14	25.9%
HIV		
n = 4	1	25.0%
C. trachomatis		
n = 50	8	16.0%
Yeasts		
n = 109	11	10.1%

Discussion

The high prevalence of HBV in homosexuals has been known for many years. The overall prevalence of HBV infection ranges from 40%-60% among homosexual men, compared with 4% to 18% among heterosexuals (1, 6). In New York 51.1% of 600 male homosexuals were found to have had past exposure to the virus as evidenced by a positive HBV-marker and with a high degree of correlation between promiscuity as well as rectal intercourse and HBV infection (7). Although fewer studies are available in heterosexuals, there is no doubt that promiscuous behaviour is a risk factor also in heterosexuals for acquiring HBV infection.

The aim of the present study was to investigate the prevalence of HBV markers in STD patients in Vienna attending two different outpatient clinics. Persons attending two outpatient clinics in the same city differed significantly in their sexual behaviour and in their marital status. Multiple episodes of STDs, promiscuous activity and the number of sexual partners during the last six months were much higher in group A, although patients of both groups had symptoms suggesting a genital infection. This fact shows that there may be great differences between STD patients not only in different countries but also in the same city. Only a low percentage of persons of group A knew about symptoms of hepatitis in themselves or about a history of hepatitis of their partner. This indicates that persons of this group were less concerned about their own health and the health conditions of their partners and furthermore the duration of the sexual companionship usually was too short to obtain knowledge about possible ailments of their sexual partners.

The prevalence of HBV was significantly different in the two STD-groups. In the 'high-risk' group 28.0% of the persons were positive for at least one HBV marker compared with 5.9% of those of group B, which may not differ from the prevalence for the general population, reported to be 4-7% (8). The comparison between a 'high-risk' and a 'low-risk' group out of the same city and investigated by identical methods makes evident that the risk of contracting HBV parallels the risk of infection with other STDs and is closely related to promiscuous behaviour. This significant association between the amount of sexual activity and the prevalence of HBV infection has also been shown in other studies (4, 9, 10). The evaluation of the different HBV markers showed a low prevalence of HBsAg positive persons in general, which was slightly higher in those of group A, but due to the small number the difference was not statistically significant. This low number of antigen-positive persons demonstrates that only few of the HBV-positive persons seem to be infectious and may therefore transmit the virus to unprotected persons.

The prevalence of HBV showed a different correlation with other STDs. Patients especially with syphilis at present or in the past had the highest risk of HBV infection. These data correlate well with other reported observations (4, 7, 11). One out of 4 patients with serological evidence of an HIV infection had also a positive HBV marker. Similar results were reported in a larger group of AIDS and pre-AIDS patients (12). So far, an interaction or association between these diseases is likely, since the mode of transmission is the same.

In summary, the results of the seroepidemiological study of HBV markers in STD patients demonstrate the significant difference of the prevalence of HBV markers between heterosexual 'high-risk' STD patients with promiscuous behaviour compared with those at low risk. Screening of STD patients should therefore include investigation for HBV markers and vaccination should be offered to those at risk.

References

1. Schreeder MT, Thompson SE, Hadler SC et al (1982) J Infect Dis 146: 7.
2. Parker HW, Varma RR, Rothwell DJ, Borkowf HI (1976) Obstet Gynecol 48: 410.
3. Blutke G (1985) Off Gesundh-Wes 47: 326.
4. Alter MJ, Antone J, Weisfuse I, Starko K, Vacalis TD, Mayhard JE (1986) JAMA 256: 1307.
5. Stary A, Kopp W, et al (1990) in press.
6. Dietzman DE, Harnish JP, Ray G, Alexander ER, Holmes KK (1977) JAMA 238: 2625.
7. Szmuness W, Much I, Prince AM et al (1975) Ann Intern Med 83: 489.
8. Szmuness W, Prince AM, Brotman B, Hirsch RL (1973) J Infect Dis 127: 17.
9. Requena-Caballero L, Vazquez-Lopez L, Arjona-Manuel C et al (1986) Med Clin (Barc) 87: 309.

10. Heun E, Whitworth B, Vogt R, Lichtenstein M, Buckley B (1987) JAMA 257: 314.
11. Baddour LM, Bucak VA, Somes G, Hudson R (1988) Sex Transm Dis 15: 174.
12. Ter Meulen J, Wittkowski KM, Kidenya JJ et al (1989) Eur J Epidemiol 5: 158.

Heterosexual transmission of hepatitis B virus

PETER PIOT, MARC VANDENBRUAENE, ERIC KEGELS AND CHRISTIAN GOILAV

Department of Microbiology, Institute of Tropical Medicine, Antwerp, Belgium

Introduction

During the 1970s several papers documented that hepatitis B virus (HBV) markers are frequently found in heterosexual men and women with multiple sex partners, and that heterosexual partners of individuals with HBV infection are at high risk for acquiring the virus (1, 2). However, for reasons that are not entirely clear, most epidemiological research and control and prevention efforts of sexually transmitted HBV have focused mainly on homosexual men.

This review discusses available evidence for the heterosexual transmission of HBV, and identifies areas for further epidemiological and operational research.

Biological basis of sexual transmission

Although the highest concentrations of HBV are found in the blood of infected individuals, HBsAg is also present in semen and vaginal secretions. HBsAg could be demonstrated in sperm in approximately half of men with HBsAg in their blood, and in most vaginal secretions (70-80%) of HBsAg seropositive women (3, 4). Intercourse during menses with an HBsAg positive woman also exposes the male partner to larger concentrations of HBV, and may be a risk factor for heterosexual HBV transmission, as demonstrated for transmission of human immunodeficiency virus (HIV) in one study (5).

In an unfortunate natural experiment, a woman became infected with HBV through artificial insemination with semen from an HBsAg carrier (6). Further experimental evidence for heterosexual transmission of HBV comes from successful infection of gibbons inoculated intravaginally with HBsAg positive semen (7).

Epidemiological studies

Support for HBV infection as a sexually transmitted disease (STD) in heterosexuals comes from several types of data, including surveillance data on hepatitis B, case control studies of hepatitis B and HBV cases, prevalence and risk factor studies in populations at risk for STDs, and sex partner and outbreak studies.

Surveillance data

Results from the Centers for Disease Control sentinel surveillance programme on acute hepatitis B suggest that at least 20 to 25% of clinical apparent hepatitis B cases in the USA acquired their infection by heterosexual intercourse (8, 9). An indepth study on risk factors for acute hepatitis B in two different areas of the USA identified heterosexual contact as the most probably source of infection in 23% of cases (10). It appears that heterosexual activity and intravenous drug use are now the leading sources of hepatitis B in the USA, with twice as many cases being acquired by heterosexual contact as compared to homosexual activity. The latter risk factor is declining, probably as a result of behavior change in response to the AIDS epidemic (8).

Early and recent data from Greece, Italy and Sweden suggest that the situation in Europe is very similar (11, 12, 43). In Sweden it is estimated that at least 50% of all hepatitis B cases are heterosexually acquired.

In addition, it is likely that a substantial proportion of cases classified as of unknown origin are infected by heterosexual contact.

Studies in populations at risk for STDs

Several surveys in Europe and North America have documented a higher prevalence rate of HBV markers among heterosexual STD patients as compared to the general population or blood donors.These surveys are summarized in Table I. As evidenced from Table I, there is a wide range of prevalence rates of HBV markers among the different studies. This may be due to a variety of factors, including differences in age, ethnic composition, socio-economic level, sex practices and level of sexual activity,

Table I HBV markers in heterosexuals with a sexually transmitted disease

City (Reference)	Year	Sex	No. tested	HBV marker positive (%)	HBV marker in control population (%)
London (Fulford et al)	1973	M	432	3	
		F	361	2	
New York City (Szmuness et al)	1975	M+F	597	24	7
Seattle (Dietzman et al)	1977	M	111	4.5	
Copenhagen (Hentzer et al)	1980	M	109	13	4
Sydney (Christopher et al)	1984	M	202	14	5
		F	200	13	
Arizona/Texas (Alter et al)	1986	M	184	8	
		F	113	8	
Barcelona (Requena Caballero et al)	1986	M	200	45	
London (Gilson et al)	1987	M		7	
		F		11	
Rome (Mele et al)	1988	M	759	42	28
Tennessee (Baddour et al)	1988	F	136	18	
Mainz (Hess et al)	1989	M+F	191	31	4
Amsterdam (Hooykaas et al)	1990	M	133	10	
		F	250	11	
Antwerp (Vandenbruaene et al)	1990	M	132	11	4
		F	71	7	
Spain (Olmos Acebos et al)	1990	M+F	441	19	
Vienna (Stary et al)	1990	M+F	461	11	
Paris (Morel et al)	1990	M+F	402	27	

and the baseline rate of HBV infection and HBV carriers in the various communities. In general, prevalence rates are higher in Southern European STD patients, reflecting a higher overall endemicity of HBV infection in Southern Europe.

Female prostitutes also yielded much higher prevalence rates of HBV markers than the general population (see Table II).

Table II HBV markers in female prostitutes who are not injecting drugs

City (reference)	Year	No. tested	HBV marker positive (%)
Cali, Columbia (Adam et al)	1974	272	25
Athens (Papaevangelou et al)	1974	293	61
Stuttgart (Frösner et al)	1975	258	33
Sydney (Christopher et al)	1984	163	31
Antwerp	1987-1989	123	18

Risk factors for HBV infection were investigated in several studies in heterosexual STD patients and in one including also university students (10, 14, 20). However, they have not been well characterized. Generally, HBV infection was significantly associated with indicators of sexual activity such as number of lifetime and of recent sex partners, a history of STD, years of sexual activity. Finally, HBsAg carriers who were found to be positive for HBeAg were significantly more likely to transmit infection to their heterosexual partners than those who were HBeAg negative (30, 31). The risk of acquiring HBV infection increased with increasing numbers of sex partners. The relative contribution of various sex practices, in particular anorectal and orogenital intercourse, to the heterosexual transmission of HBV is unclear. Heterosexuals with syphilis or serological markers of syphilis have usually much higher prevalence rates of HBV markers (17). The reason for this association is not clear, but the unintentional inclusion of homosexual and bisexual men among groups of heterosexual STD patients may be one explanation.

Studies of partners and of outbreaks

It was the observation of acute hepatitis B among spouses, and sex partners of HBV carriers that provided the first evidence of sexual transmission of what used to be called 'serum hepatitis' (32). Subsequently, several studies have documented that between one-third and half of both female and male heterosexual partners of patients with hepatitis B or of chronic HBsAg carriers show evidence of past or present infection (2, 30, 33-36).

Interestingly, HBV prevalence appears to be higher in male partners of infected women than vice versa, leading several authors to conclude that female to male transmission of HBV is more efficient than male to female transmission. However, this needs confirmation in prospective studies which control for known risk factors for sexual transmission of HBV. The risk of transmission during a single episode of sexual intercourse is not well known, but may be substantial in the presence of risk factors such as HBeAg and vaginal bleeding (37).

Investigations of clusters of acute hepatitis B have also documented heterosexual spread of HBV infection (37-41).

The combined data clearly suggest that the risk of HBV infection in heterosexuals with multiple sex partners may reach a level similar to that in homosexual men with comparable promiscuity. Reasons for overall higher infection rates in homosexual men as compared with heterosexuals may include a higher frequency of anorectal intercourse (a major risk factor for HBV transmission in gay men), a larger average number of sex partners, and a higher rate of HBsAg carriage.

Conclusion and research needs

The available data all indicate an important role for heterosexual activity in the spread of HBV. In order to strengthen and rationalize control efforts against HBV infection in heterosexuals, further research is necessary on questions such as: 1) what is the population attributable risk of heterosexual transmission for HBV infection in the industrialized world and in developing countries; 2) what is the rate of female-to-male and of male-to-female transmission of HBV; 3) what are specific risk factors for heterosexual transmission of HBV in various populations, and by gender; 4) what is the source of infection in HBV cases presently classified as of unknown transmission category; 5) what is the impact of AIDS prevention activities on HBV incidence in various populations; 6) what are the most efficient/effective methods to deliver HBV-vaccine in heterosexual populations? (42).

However, present knowledge, and the severity of hepatitis B and its sequelae amply justify public health intervention without waiting for the results of the proposed research.

References

1. Fulford KWM, Dane DS, Catterall RD, Woof R, Denning JV (1973) Lancet i: 1470.
2. Szmuness W, Much MI, Prince AM et al (1975) Ann Intern Med 83: 489.
3. Heathcote J, Cameron CH, Dane DS (1974) Lancet 1: 71.
4. Parker HW, Varma RR, Rothwell DJ, Barkwf HI (1976) Obstet Gynecol 48: 410.
5. De Vincenzi I, Ancelle-Park RA, Brunet JB (1989) Brit Med J 298: 411.
6. Berry WR, Gotterfeld RL, Alter HJ, Vierling JM (1987) JAMA 257: 1079.
7. Scott RM, Snitbahn R, Bancroft WH, Alter HJ, Tingpalapong (1980) J Infect Dis 142: 67.
8. Centers for Disease Control (1988) MMWR 37: 429.
9. Alter MJ, Hadler SC, Margolis HS, Alexander WJ, Hu PY, Judson FN, Mares A, Miller JK, Moyer LA (1990) JAMA 263: 1218.
10. Alter MJ, Coleman PJ, Alexander J, Kramer E, Miller JK, Mandel E, Hadler SC, Margolis NS (1989) JAMA 262: 1201.
11. Papaevangelou G, Roumeliotou-Karayannis A, Tassopoulos N, Kolaitis N, Stathopoulou P (1983) J Infect Dis 147: 987.
12. Pasquini P, Mele A, Stazi AM (1990) This volume.
13. Dietzman DE, Harnisch JP, Ray CG, Alexander ER, Holmes KK (1977) JAMA 238: 2625.
14. Hentzer B, Skinhoj P, Hoybye G, Nielsen AO, Kvorning SA, Faber V (1980) Scand J Infect Dis 12: 245.
15. Christopher PJ, Mailer PT, Crewe EB, Murphy AM (1984) Aust NZ J Med 14: 491.
16. Alter MJ, Ahtone J, Weisfuse I et al (1986) JAMA 256: 1307.
17. Requena Caballero L, Vazquez Lopez F, Arjona Manuel C, Romero Guerrero J, Casado Jiminez M (1986) Med Clin (Barcelona) 87: 309.
18. Gilson RJC, De Ruiter A, Waite J, Loveday C, Kelly G, Weller IVD (1990) This volume.
19. Mele A, Franco E, Caprilli F, Gentilli G, Stazi MA, Zaratti L, Cpitanio B, Crescimbeni E, Corona R, Pana A, Pasquini P (1988) Eur J Epidemiol 4: 488.

20. Baddour LM, Bucak VA, Somes G, Hudson R (1988) Sex Transm Dis 15: 174.
21. Hooykaas C, Coutinho RA, van Doornum GJJ (1990) This volume.
22. Vandenbruaene M, Goeman J, Avonts D, Vranckx R, Piot P. Unpublished.
23. Hess G, Massing A, Rossof S, Voth R, Schütt H, Clemens R, Meyer zum Büschenfelde KH (1989) Lancet 2: 987.
24. Olmos L, Vilata JL, Rodriguez Pichardo A (1990) This volume.
25. Stary A, Kopp W, Vitouch C (1990) This volume.
26. Morel P, Morinet F, Janier M, Lassau F, Meouchy R, Perol Y (1990) This volume.
27. Adam E, Hollinger FB, Melnick JL, Duenas A, Rawls WE (1974) J Infect Dis 129: 317.
28. Papaevangelou G, Trichopoulos T, Kremastinou T et al (1974) Br Med J 2: 256.
29. Frösner GG, Buchholz HM, Gerth HJ (1975) Am J Epidemiol 102: 241.
30. Bernier RH, Sampliner R, Gerety R, Tabor E, Hamilton F, Nathanson N (1982) Am J Epidemiol 116: 199.
31. Perrillo RP, Gelb L, Campbell C et al (1979) Gastroenterology 76: 1319.
32. Hersch T, Melnick JL, Goyal RK, Hollinger FB (1971) N Engl J Med 285: 1363.
33. Redeker AG, Mosley JW, Gocke DJ et al (1975) N Engl J Med 293: 1055.
34. Inaba N, Ohkawa R, Matsuura A, Kudoh J, Takamizawa H (1979) Br J Vener Dis 55: 366.
35. Papaevangelou G, Tassopoulos N, Roumeliotou-Karayanmis A, Richardson SC (1985) J Infect Dis 152: 231.
36. Ko YC, Yen YY, Yeh SM, Lan SJ (1989) J Med Virol 27: 142.
37. Clee WB, Hunter PR (1987) Br Med J 295: 530.
38. Heun E, Whitworth B, Vogt R, Lichtenstein M, Buckley B (1987) JAMA 257: 314.
39. Fagan EA, Smith FP, Davison F, Williams R (1986) Lancet 2: 538.
40. Gordon SC,Reobly KR, Jeffers LJ, Schiff ER(1985) South Med J 78: 1142.
41. Wright RA (1975) JAMA 232: 717.
42. World Health Organization (1990) Geneva, World Health Organization, WHO/VDT.
43. Böttinger M, Christenson B (1990) This volume.

HEPATITIS B PREVENTION STRATEGIES

Hepatitis B: A sexually transmitted disease in heterosexuals.
P. Piot and F.E. Andre, editors

Prevention of the transmission of hepatitis B infection by the sexual route

F.E. Andre

SmithKline Beecham Biologicals, 89 rue de l'Institut, 1330 Rixensart, Belgium

Introduction

Much has been learned about the epidemiology and biology of the hepatitis B virus (HBV) since the discovery of the Australia antigen by Blumberg and coworkers (1,2). Originally thought to be transmitted solely by blood or blood-derived products, it is now known that infectious virus can be present in other body fluids such as saliva, tears, sweat, semen and vaginal secretions.

Evidence that hepatitis B infection can be transmitted by body fluids, especially through sexual contact, has been obtained in studies describing cases of infection among spouses and sexual partners of individuals with acute hepatitis B or known HBV carriers (3-7). A high prevalence of hepatitis B markers has also been found in the sera of prostitutes (8,9), sexually-active homosexual men (10,11) and individuals with a history of other sexually transmitted diseases (12,13). Homosexual men have long been considered at high risk of infection, but an increase in the use of condoms due to an awareness of other sexually transmissible diseases such as AIDS has lowered the incidence of hepatitis B in these individuals (14). An important rise in the frequency of hepatitis B has been demonstrated following heterosexual contact, which accounted for nearly one-fifth of all cases of hepatitis B reported in the four sentinel counties in the USA during 1987 (15).

Prevention of infection with HBV

Although 'safe' behaviour, i.e. the use of condoms and restriction of sexual activity, and passive immunization with hepatitis B immunoglobulin can effectively guard against infection, the protection these measures provide is only temporary. Active immunization, affording durable immunity, is clearly the most practical method of preventing hepatitis B infection and chronic carriage of HBV. Until recently, only plasma-derived vaccines (PDV), manufactured using the hepatitis B surface antigen (HBsAg) purified from the plasma of chronic carriers, were available. For several reasons, their use had not been extensive. These vaccines are relatively expensive in comparison with other vaccines, due to the limited supply of HBsAg-positive plasma, a long production cycle, and the need for extensive testing using animals such as chimpanzees. In addition, the unfounded fear that human pathogenic organisms (especially the human immunodeficiency virus, refs. 16, 17) could be spread by the vaccines discouraged their use. Advances in recombinant DNA technology permitted the development of vaccines, using the surface antigen expressed in yeast cells (18, 19).

These techniques allow the manufacture of virtually unlimited quantities of yeast-derived vaccine (YDV) which are free from potential human pathogens.

Techniques used in the production of YDV

The gene coding for the HBsAg of an adw_2 serotype of HBV was isolated and then cloned in baker's yeast, *Saccharomyces cerevisiae*. The protein is expressed, extracted from the yeast culture, and purified in the form of 22 nm particles using ultrafiltration and chromatographic techniques (19). The yeast-derived HBsAg is biochemically, physically and immunologically similar to the non-glycosylated form of the surface antigen found in human plasma (19, 20). The purified particles are formulated into a vaccine (Engerix-B®, SmithKline Beecham Biologicals, Rixensart, Belgium) by adsorbtion onto aluminium hydroxide.

Clinical experience with the YDV

After extensive *in vitro* and *in vivo* preclinical testing, clinical trials were initiated in human volunteers. Since February 1984, 135 clinical studies have been carried out world-wide. They have involved over 17,500 volunteers of all ages in representative population groups likely to require vaccination. These trials have demonstrated the safety and low reactogenicity of the YDV; the most frequently reported symptom after vaccine administration in adults has been shown to be mild soreness at the site of injection (21). The primary safety concern with the YDV, i.e. the possibility of induction of hypersensitivity to yeast proteins, has been shown to be unfounded (19, 22). Post-marketing surveillance following commercial distribution of more than 18 million doses of this vaccine has confirmed these findings.

Comparative studies using commercial lots of PDV have shown that the YDV induces antibodies which are virtually identical to those observed after administration of PDV with regard to epitope specificity and avidity (20). The persistence of anti-HBs with time is also similar for the two types of vaccines (23, 24). YDV can be used to boost antibody titres in subjects who have been primed with a PDV (23, 25).

The protective efficacy of the YDV has been assessed in studies in homosexual men (26) and mentally handicapped patients (27). These trials have shown that the annual incidence of HB infection decreased following vaccination to virtually zero from historical rates of approximately 12% and 9%, respectively. Other clinical trials have been carried out in neonates of HBe antigen-positive carrier mothers, who have a risk of between 65% to 90% of becoming chronic carriers (28-30). It has been shown previously that rapid prophylaxis with hepatitis B immunoglobulin following birth can decrease the carrier rate in these infants to approximately 30% (31, 32). When 10 μg doses of the YDV were administered to a group of high-risk infants at birth, 1, 2 and 12 months of age, only 3.4% (2/58) of those infants treated became chronically infected with the HBV (33).

Factors which may influence antibody titres in vaccinees

Vaccination schedule

The immunogenicity of the YDV has been assessed following administration of the vaccine according to different schedules. Two three-dose schedules are currently advised; 0, 1, 2 months and 0, 1, 6 months. The seroconversion rates following administration of the three vaccine doses to healthy adults are above 95% for both schedules, although antibody titres are higher when the latter schedule is used. The overall results on over 3000 subjects (approximately 1700 on each schedule) are shown in Figure 1. One month after the third vaccine dose, the GMT of subjects on the former schedule was 139 mlU/ml; the GMT for individuals vaccinated according to a 0, 1, 6 month schedule was equal to 1190 mlU/ml at month 7.

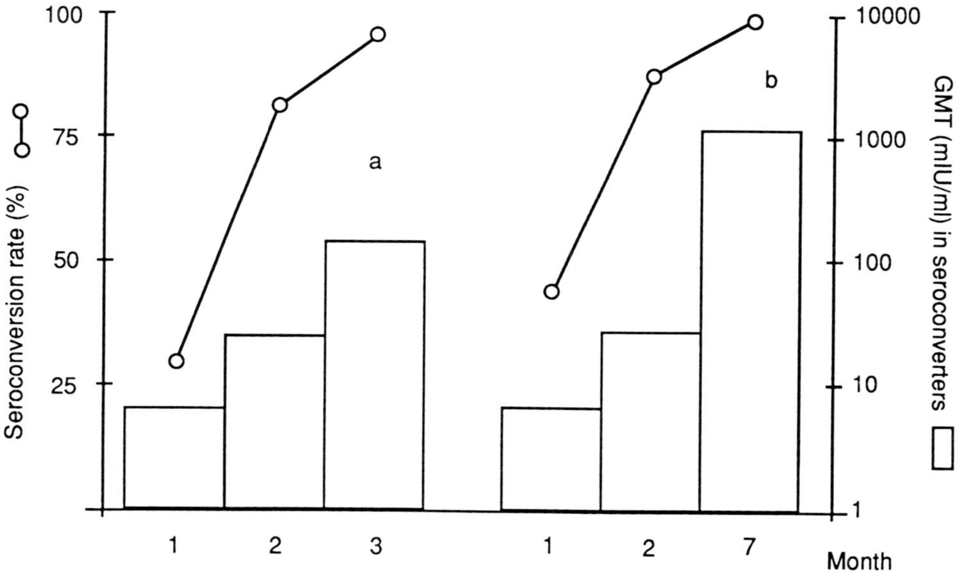

Fig. 1. Seroconversion rates and geometric mean anti-HBs titres (GMT) in healthy adults vaccinated with 20 g doses of YDV according to either a 0, 1, 2 month schedule (a) or a 0, 1, 6 month schedule (b).

The administration of the third dose of vaccine at month 2 rather than month 6 will give, however, a more rapid increase in anti-HBs titres; this schedule is therefore to be prefered when protection against infection is rapidly required, e.g. for neonates of HBeAg-positive carrier mothers, for travellers going from areas of low to high endemicity, or for STD patients.

An additional reason for the use of this schedule, especially in high-risk settings, is the problem of vaccinee compliance. Table 1 gives the number of adult vaccinees enrolled in the clinical trials who complete the entire vaccination course for the two vaccination schedules. Whereas more than 95% of these individuals returned for the third dose at month 2, 87% returned when this dose was given at month 6. Similar drop-out rates have also been reported by others (34, 35). It is generally accepted that compliance will be lower under 'field conditions' than in a clinical trial, making the 0, 1, 2 month schedule preferable when vaccinee compliance may be questionnable.

Table I Vaccinee compliance in healthy adults according to the schedule used for vaccination

Vaccination schedule (month)	Number of subjects given first dose	Number of subjects given third dose	Compliance (%)
0, 1, 2	2308	2201	95.4
0, 1, 6	2197	1907	86.8

Vaccine dose level

Initial dose-range studies performed in young healthy adults demonstrated a trend towards a dose-related anti-HBs response. In order to evoke an immune response similar to that induced by the PDVs, a vaccine dose level of 20 μg was chosen for adults. This level gives seroconversion rates greater than 95%, independently of the vaccination schedule used (Figure 1). In addition, although seroconversion rates are similar for lower doses of vaccine after the full vaccination course, a greater proportion of subjects seroconvert after only two 20 μg doses as compared to either 5 μg or 10 μg (Figure 2). It is therefore better to give higher doses of vaccine when vaccinee compliance may be low. A 20 μg dose will also provide a 'safety margin' to ensure adequate antibody levels in 'poor responders' and compensate for any loss of potency during shipment and storage.

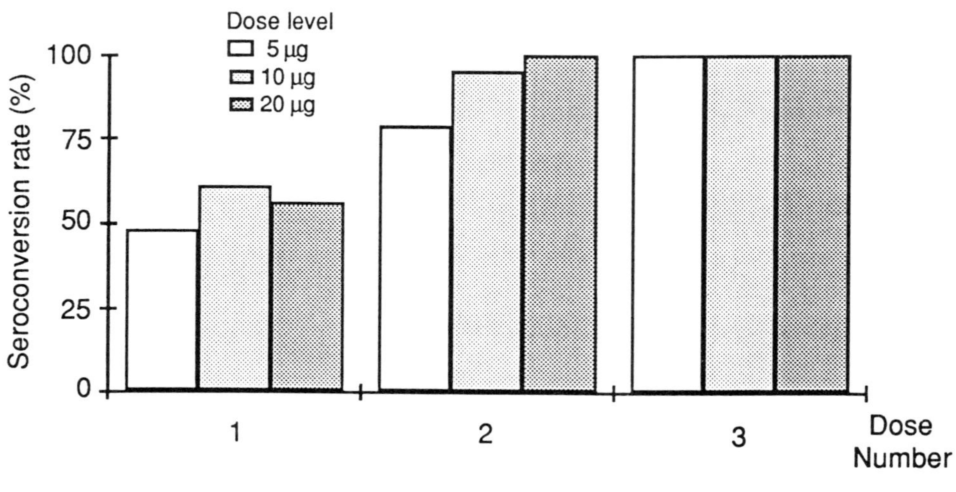

Fig. 2. Seroconversion rates after vaccination of young healthy adults with YDV at different dose levels according to a 0, 1, 2 month vaccination schedule. Antibody titres were measured one month after each vaccine dose.

Conclusions

The clinical studies with the YDV in a large range of representative populations have shown that this vaccine is safe and is well tolerated. These results have been confirmed by post-marketing surveillance of the over 18 million commercially distributed doses.

The YDV has been shown to be highly immunogenic, inducing seroconversion in over 95% of all subjects vaccinated, regardless of the vaccination schedule used. Its effectiveness in the prevention of hepatitis B infection has been shown in three groups of individuals at high-risk; homosexual men, the institutionalised mentally handicapped and neonates of HBeAg-positive carrier mothers.

The 20 μg dose level is recommended for adults as it may help to compensate for poor vaccinee compliance or for a decrease in immune response in 'poor responders'. It will also provide a 'safety margin' against potential loss of vaccine potency during shipment or storage.

The widespread use of the YDV in the protection of subjects at risk of hepatitis B due to their sexual behaviour should have a significant impact on virus transmission.

References

1. Blumberg BS, Alter HJ, Visnich S (1965) JAMA 191: 541.
2. Blumberg BS, Gerstley BJS, Hungerford DA, London WT, Sutnick AI (1967) Ann Intern Med 66: 924.
3. Hersh T, Melnick J L, Goyal RK et al (1971) N Engl J Med 285: 1363.
4. Heathcote J, Gateau P, Sherlock S (1974) Lancet i: 370.
5. Redeker AG, Mosley JW, Gocke DJ, McKee AP, Pollack W (1975) N Engl J Med 293: 1055.
6. Ko YC, Yen YY, Yeh SM, Lan SJ (1989) J Med Virol 27: 142.
7. Struve J, Giesecke J, Lindh G, Weiland O (1990) J Infect 20: 111.
8. Papaevangelou G, Trichopoulos T, Kremastinou T, et al (1974) Brit Med J 2: 256.
9. Frösner GG, Buchholz HM, Gerth HJ (1975) Am J Epidemiol 102: 241.
10. Szmuness W, Stevens CE, Harley EJ et al (1980) N Engl J Med 303: 833.
11. Hentzer B, Skinhøj P, Hoybye G, Nielsen AO, Kvørning SA, Faber V (1980) Scand J Infect Dis 12: 245.
12. Ter Meulen J, Wittkowski KM, Kidenya JJ et al (1989) Eur J Epidemiol 5: 158.
13. Rosenblum LS, Hadler SC, Castro KG, Lieb S, Jaffe HW and the Belle Glade Study Group (1990) J Infect Dis 161: 407.
14. Alter MJ, Hadler SC, Margolis HS et al (1990) JAMA 263: 1218.
15. Anonymous (1988) MMWR 37: 429.
16. Barré-Sinoussi F, Nugeyre MT, Girard M, Tron F, Chermann JC (1985) Lancet i: 274.
17. Dienstag JL, Werner BG, McLane MF et al (1985) JAMA 254: 1064.
18. McALeer WJ, Bunyak EB, Maigetter RZ, Wampler DE, Miller WJ, Hilleman MR (1984) Nature 307: 178.
19. Pêtre J, Van Wijnendaele F, De Neys B, et al (1987) Postgrad Med J 63 (suppl 2): 73.
20. Hauser P, Voet P, Simoen E et al (1987) Postgrad Med J 63 (suppl 2): 83.
21. André FE (1990) Vaccine 8 (suppl March): 574
22. Wiedermann G, Scheiner O, Ambrosch F et al (1988) Int Arch Allergy Appl Immunol 85: 130.
23. Just M, Berger R, Scheiermann N (1988) Vaccine 6: 401.
24. Scheiermann N, Gesemann M, Maurer C, Just M, Berger R (1990) Vaccine 8 (suppl March): S44.

25. Ambrosch F, Kremsner P, Weidermann G et al (1986) Lancet i: 1101.
26. Goilav C, Prinsen H, Piot P (1990) Vaccine 8 (suppl March): S50.
27. Van Damme P, Vrankx R, Safary A, André FE, Meheus A (1987) Am J Med 87(3A): 26S.
28. Wong VCW, Ip HMH, Reesink HW et al (1984) Lancet i: 921.
29. Xu ZY, Liu CB, Francis DP et al (1985) Pediatrics 76: 713.
30. Pongpipat D, Suvatte V, Assateerawatts A (1986) Asian Pac J Allergy Immunol 4: 33.
31. Beasley RP, Hwang LY, Stevens CE et al (1983) Hepatology 3: 135.
32. Ko TM, Lin KH, Ho MM et al (1987) J Med Virol 21: 301.
33. Poovorawan Y, Sanpavat S, Pongpunlert W, Chumdermpadetsuk S, Sentrakul P, Safary A (1989) JAMA 261: 3278.
34. Francis DP, Hadler SC, Thompson SE et al (1982) Ann Intern Med 97: 362.
35. Fagan EA, Tolley P, Smith HM et al (1987) J Med Virol 21: 49.

© 1990 Elsevier Science Publishers B.V. (Biomedical Division)
Hepatitis B: A sexually transmitted disease in heterosexuals.
P. Piot and F.E. Andre, editors

Hepatitis B in 1990 – Where are we and where are we going? The WHO programme for control of viral hepatitis

Mark A. Kane, Yuri Ghendon, Paul-Henri Lambert

Microbiology and Immunology Support Services, Division of Communicable Diseases, World Health Organization, 1211 Geneva 27, Switzerland

Introduction

Hepatitis B, one of the major diseases of mankind, is now preventable with a safe and effective vaccine, the first vaccine against cancer. More than 2000 million individuals have been infected with the hepatitis B virus (HBV) globally, of whom some 280 million are chronically infected carriers of this virus. These carriers are at high risk of serious illness and death from cirrhosis of the liver and primary liver cancer, diseases that kill one to two million carriers per year. Primary liver cancer caused by HBV infection is one of the top three causes of cancer death in much of Africa, Asia, and the Pacific Basin. In addition, these carriers constitute a reservoir of infected individuals who perpetuate the infection from generation to generation.

Most people in Africa, Eastern and Southeast Asia, the Pacific Basin, the Amazon Basin, and parts of the Middle East become infected with this virus during childhood, either from an infected mother (perinatal transmission), or from child-to-child transmission. Infection during childhood is especially likely to lead to the chronic carrier state. In Europe, North America, much of Latin America, and Australia hepatitis B infection is a major sexually transmitted disease and a significant cause of morbidity for health care personnel and certain other groups defined by lifestyle and occupation.

Hepatitis B (HB) vaccine, if given prior to infection, can prevent disease and the carrier state from developing in almost all individuals. The vaccine is most effectively used as a routine part of the infant immunization schedule, although it can be used at any age. Recent dramatic decreases in vaccine cost (from U.S. $50 to U.S. $3—$6 per pediatric series) have allowed public health officials to consider the mass use of this vaccine in infant immunization programmes, although it is still considerably more expensive than the other routine childhood vaccines. Many countries, especially in Asia, the Pacific Basin, and Middle East have begun extensive infant immunization programmes, and there is tremendous interest in starting such programmes worldwide.

The WHO programme for control of viral hepatitis

The Microbiology and Immunology Support Services (MIM) section of the Division of Communicable Diseases (CDS) has been actively involved in hepatitis B control efforts for many years through its Programme for the Control of Viral Hepatitis, the Technical Advisory Group (TAG) on Viral Hepatitis, and the network of Collaborating Centers for Reference and Research on Viral Hepatitis.

During 1989-90 efforts to control hepatitis B were greatly increased:

* A full time position for viral hepatitis was created and filled.
* A contribution of one million doses of hepatitis B vaccine was received from a major vaccine manufacturer to allow expanded programme activities, and commitments from several other vaccine producers have been received.
* Control projects in Brazil, Cameroon, Gabon, Mongolia, and Jordan have been established.
* Projects are in the discussion stage for programmes in Peru, Lesotho, Botswansa, Cuba and several other countries.
* Close collaboration has been established with the EPI to provide the technical input necessary for the integration of HB vaccine into the EPI.
* WHO and the United Nations Children's Fund (UNICEF) will attempt to reduce the cost of HB vaccine through large scale purchases by UNICEF.
* HB control efforts are being coordinated with other programmes and activities involved in areas of mutual interest. These include WHO programmes on: sexually transmitted diseases, safe blood supply, biologicals, aids, drug dependence, occupational health, and reagent development. Agencies outside of WHO include the International Task Force on Hepatitis B Immunization, the International Agency for Research on Cancer, and the International Atomic Energy Agency.
* Operational research activities to answer practical questions about HB immunization is underway in our demonstration projects, with our collaborating centres, and with EPI. Projects are examining the issues of optimal vaccine schedules, duration of immunity, vaccine interactions, combined vaccines, freezing point and vaccine stability, and cost effectiveness.
* Applied research on vaccine development is underway in the WHO Trans-Disease Vaccinology Programme. Development is underway on a pulse release polymer coated antigen that may lead to a single dose HB vaccine.

1990 – Where are we?

The November 1989 EPI/CDS Update entitled 'Hepatitis B Vaccine: Attacking a Pandemic' reported the current global situation with respect to hepatitis B vaccine. A total of 22 countries, primarily in the Western Pacific and Eastern Mediterranean Regions have a policy of vaccinating all newborns with HB vaccine or plan to do so this year. Twenty three additional countries have pilot infant immunization projects underway in selected regions of the country or plan to begin such projects this year. Twenty seven other countries have selective immunization programmes in place or planned. Selective programmes may include screening of pregnant women and vaccination of newborns of carrier mothers, immunization of health care personnel, and/or immunization of other high risk groups.

The single most important step in the global control of hepatitis B will be the integration of this vaccine into the EPI. The EPI is a network of international, regional, national, and local immunization programmes that reaches to the village level and is largely responsible for the fact that about two thirds of the world's children are vaccinated, a truly remarkable achievement. The integration of HB vaccine was recommended by the Technical Advisory Group on Viral Hepatitis and the Global Advisory Group of EPI in 1987, and strongly reiterated in 1989. The EPI has greatly increased its activities on hepatitis B over the last year, and there is every indication that they are rapidly moving toward integration of HB vaccine into their system.

Where do vaccines come from in the developing world? In some of the larger countries, at least some of the vaccines are produced nationally. In some of the wealthier developing countries, vaccines produced elsewhere are purchased. Frequent use is made of the reimbursable facility offered by UNICEF, or, in the Region of the Americas, the Pan American Health Organization rotating fund for vaccine purchase. But in the majority of developing countries, the vaccines are donated. For vaccines used in the EPI, UNICEF is the major provider, supplemented by donations from bilateral development agencies. At present, Rotary International, through donations to UNICEF is a major provider of polio vaccines.

Vaccine price remains an important impediment to widespread use in developing countries. Countries outside of Europe, North America, and Australia are able to obtain HB vaccine for public sector programmes for U.S. $0.90 to $2.00 per pediatric dose. Although this represents a dramatic improvement over the $20 per pediatric dose price of a few years ago, $2.7 to $6 per child is more than UNICEF pays for BCG, OPV, DPT, and measles vaccine combined. Introduction of HB vaccine at current prices would more than double the cost for infant vaccines in many parts of the world (money that many governments, UNICEF, and other international agencies do not have) and money that most donors have not yet been willing to give.

WHO and UNICEF have held discussions about the possibility of UNICEF procuring HB vaccine in an attempt to develop a global revolving fund for hepatitis B vaccine. UNICEF has agreed to do this if donors can be found to purchase the vaccine, or if countries who wish to purchase vaccine ask UNICEF to do the procurement. Pooling of orders from a number of countries and competitive bidding with large orders should lead to significantly lower prices, which in turn would allow more countries to afford HB immunization. UNICEF procurement would also insure that participating countries received vaccine that meets WHO requirements, and that uniform shipping and storage conditions are met. The Pan American Health Organization (PAHO) revolving fund could serve a similar function for the Americas.

HBV control strategies in areas of 'high' and 'intermediate' endemicity

It is now generally recognized that universal infant immunization with HB vaccine is the basic strategy for long term control of hepatitis B in areas of 'high' and 'intermediate' endemicity. Infection during infancy and early childhood plays a disproportionate role in generating the HBV carrier pool, and in much of the world the infant immunization programmes are the only functioning vaccine delivery systems. Countries with additional resources may wish to add additional programmes once infant immunization is established. These programmes may include 'catch up' immunization of older children, maternal screening and treatment of infants of carrier mothers with HBIG and HB vaccine, and immunization of health care workers and other 'high risk' groups.

HBV control strategies in areas of 'low endemicity'

North America, Western Europe, Australia, and parts of South America are considered to be areas of 'low endemicity'. In these areas perinatal and child-to-child transmission is relatively uncommon, and most infections occur in adults through sexual activity, needle sharing during drug abuse, or during occupational exposure to blood. Since the availability of HB vaccine in 1981-82, strategies for HBV control have stressed the immunization of 'high risk' groups, and the screening of pregnant women and treatment of the infants of HBV carrier mothers. There is now serious doubt that this strategy will lead to the control of hepatitis B.

With few exceptions the impact of this strategy has been the immunization of health care workers and persons in institutions for the developmentally disabled – about 85% of HB vaccine sold in the U.S. and Europe has been used in these groups. Although it is certainly good medical practice to immunize these individuals, cases in health care workers represent less that 5% of reported cases of HB in the U.S. Intravenous drug abusers, those who acquire HBV infection through homosexual or heterosexual activity, and those who belong to ethnic minorities where HBV infection is prevalent are difficult to access and are often infected before they present to any health setting where immunization could be offered. For these reasons immunization of all infants, and possibly adolescent immunization for an interim period is being proposed by a number of experts as the only strategy that will provide long term control of HBV infection even in areas of 'low' prevalence.

Goals

Global control of hepatitis B is within our reach. WHO will be working toward the following goals:

* Universal infant HB immunization through complete integration into the EPI.
* Vaccine price proportional to other EPI antigens.
* Development of a Global Revolving Fund for vaccine procurement.
* Appropriate local production of HB vaccine through transfer of technology.
* Universal HBsAg screening of blood and blood products.
* Appropriate local production and distribution of hepatitis reagents.
* Immunization for occupational exposure and high risk lifestyles.
* Development of 'secondary prevention' strategies for HBV carriers. This would include effective anti-viral chemotherapy and determination of the efficacy of alpha fetoprotein screening for early detection of liver cancer.
* Development of HB vaccines that are effective with a single injection and are stable outside the cold chain.

Conclusion

HB vaccines have proven themselves to be stable, safe, immunogenic, and effective. There are no technical or scientific impediments to their immediate use. Indeed, the dimensions of the global problem of HBV infection make it clear that their use is a matter of urgency. As with all vaccines, research and development efforts must continue to improve the vaccine and its preparations, determine the most cost effective strategies for delivering it, and lower the vaccine cost. The final task before us is to develop national programmes and obtain financial resources to provide this important antigen to the world's children.

© 1990 Elsevier Science Publishers B.V. (Biomedical Division)
Hepatitis B: A sexually transmitted disease in heterosexuals.
P. Piot and F.E. Andre, editors

Control of sexual transmission of hepatitis B virus infections

FRANKLYN N. JUDSON

Programme of Sexually Transmitted Diseases, World Health Organization, 1211 Geneva 27, Switzerland

Prior to the AIDS epidemic, more than 50% of new hepatitis B virus (HBV) infections in developed North American and European countries were sexually transmitted; approximately one quarter by heterosexual men and women and one third by homosexual men (1). The percentage of HBV infections attributable to heterosexual transmission in developing countries and in developed countries of Asia is unknown but probably is proportionate to the percent of the population which escapes perinatal and early childhood infection.

As reported by Dr M Kane the ultimate control of hepatitis B in areas of 'high' and 'intermediate' endemicity will depend upon universal immunization of infants with hepatitis B vaccine. This strategy acknowledges the fact that infant immunization programmes are the only functioning vaccine delivery systems in much of the world and that most infections occur during infancy and early childhood. Universal immunization of infants, perhaps followed by booster doses of hepatitis B vaccine in early adolescence, would eliminate the need for any other programmes to control sexual transmission of hepatitis B virus (HBV) infections in these populations.

In developed countries with low hepatitis B endemicity rates, infection of infants is uncommon and a large majority of all cases occur in sexually active young and middle aged men and women. As a result, and based primarily upon cost/effectiveness considerations, control strategies thus far have centered on identification of individuals with high risk sexual lifestyles for behavioural interventions and selective immunization with hepatitis B vaccine.

I will review some of the practical experiential and epidemiological realities of this approach which cast substantial doubt on whether it ever can succeed. My conclusions are heavily weighted by studies from the United States which may not be generalizable to other developed countries with different socioeconomic and ethnic make-ups.

In contrast to universal childhood immunization, precisely targeted programmes to control sexually transmitted diseases (STD) in adults must be designed around a thorough understanding of the epidemiology and natural history of infection, known routes of transmission, and easily identifiable measures of risk. In the case of sexually transmitted hepatitis B, much of this information is still lacking.

Sexual transmission of hepatitis B was first extensively studied in homosexual men attending metropolitan STD clinics (3). They were found to have prevalence rates of current and prior HBV infection in the order of 20 to 30 times those of age matched heterosexual men (4). Although studies indicated that infection was highly associated with active oral, anal and passive anogenital contact, and that the ano-rectum, which often contained punctate bleeding spots (5), could serve as both a source and portal of entry for HBV, the relative and absolute efficiencies of different types of sexual contact were never determined. These fine points aside, a cohort study performed just prior to the first reports of a new acquired immunodeficiency syndrome (AIDS) in homosexual men in 1981, calculated frighteningly high annual HBV infection rates (incidence) of 15-20% in seronegative men (Centers for Disease Control, unpublished).

Although the first and largest controlled studies of the efficacy of hepatitis B vaccine appropriately were performed in high risk homosexual men (6), the vaccine never was effectively used to control sexually transmitted hepatitis B. As noted by others, of an estimated 2.5 million persons who have received hepatitis B vaccine, 80-85%, were health care workers or institutionalized developmentally disabled individuals who account for less than 5% of all reported cases of hepatitis B and play almost no role in perpetuating endemic infection levels. The failure to mount large scale hepatitis B control programmes for homosexual men was multifactorial and included high cost of vaccine, inadequate understanding of the long term complications of hepatitis B by both homosexual men and health care providers, the desire for sexual orientation anonymity and the passive nature of most vaccination efforts.

Nonetheless, and owing almost entirely to major reductions in high risk sexual activity by homosexual men in response to the deadly AIDS epidemic, incidence rates of gonorrhoea, syphilis and hepatitis B have fallen dramatically since the early 1980's. For the period 1982-85 homosexual men experienced 21% of all hepatitis B reported through the Centers for Disease Controls' Sentinel Counties Surveillance Study, or more than one third of all cases with a known source. By 1988 hepatitis B attributable to male homosexual exposure had declined to 7.2% (1).

Future hepatitis B control programmes targeted at homosexual men must take this trend into account as well as the obvious implications of a concurrent AIDS epidemic i.e. a homosexual man given hepatitis B vaccine because of continuing high risk sexual activity will probably die of AIDS before any of the long term complications of hepatitis B virus infection can develop. Cost/effectiveness of a new vaccine initiative would be further reduced for men already infected with human immunodeficiency virus as a consequence of lower anti-HBs seroconversion rates and geometric mean titers, higher HBV carriage rates if infected during vaccination (7), possible stimulation of lymphocytes to produce HIV, and the likelihood of dying of AIDS before vaccine benefit is realized.

It would seem that limited funds for vaccination of homosexual men against hepatitis B would be better spent in modifying residual high risk sexual behaviour which is the common denominator for all sexually transmitted diseases, including AIDS.

With the decline in the fraction of hepatitis B attributable to homosexual men, attention has shifted to sexual transmission among heterosexual men and women, which according to the CDC's Sentinel Counties Study, comprised 26% of all cases in 1988 (1). This fraction probably is significantly underestimated because a large portion of the 37% with 'no known source' likely was sexually transmitted. Supporting evidence includes: 1) an age-incidence distribution suggestive of sexual transmission, 2) a mutually exclusive hierarchical risk assignment method which favours parenteral drug use over sexual transmission, 3) a restrictive definition which requires for heterosexual attribution sexual contact with a known HBV infection or more than one sexual partner within 6 months, and 4) a prevalence of HBV markers of 19% in household and sexual contacts of hepatitis B patients with no identifiable source for infection, compared with 4% to 7% in the general population (1).

The actual routes of HBV heterosexual transmission, as well as their relative and absolute efficiencies remain largely unknown. Little new information has been reported since 1981 when I reviewed the 'Epidemiology of Sexually Transmitted Hepatitis B Infections in Heterosexuals' (8). The highest concentration of HBsAg is found in blood; but HBsAg also appears in saliva, semen, menstrual discharge, vaginal secretions, faeces, urine and tears. Saliva is the secretion most often mentioned as a potential vehicle for transmitting HBV. Infectious saliva could provide a common explanation for the high rates of secondary infection observed in siblings and mothers of leukemic children with hepatitis B, in children fed premasticated food by HBV carrier mothers, and in heterosexual contacts of patients with hepatitis B.

If HBV infection in heterosexuals is predominantly transmitted by vaginal intercourse, the endocervix, endometrium, cervical ectopy, and cervical infection with other STDs provide biologically plausible exposed vascular targets for the low concentrations of HBV found in semen. Also, 5-10% of women in developed countries occasionally practice anorectal intercourse, adding vascular rectal mucosa as another target. In the absence of high prevalence rates of genital ulcer disease in men, one might anticipate higher prevalence and incidence rates of HBV infections in women. In this regard, when gender specific incidence rates per 100,000 population are computed for the Sentinel Counties Study period of 1986-88, respective rates for cases in heterosexual women and men are a near identical 3.0 and 2.9 (1), a parity not found with most genital STDs.

Given that 1) oral contact may be an important route of transmission; 2) most heterosexual cases do not report large numbers of partners; 3) fewer than 25% of cases can identify a known infected contact; and, 4) as many as 75% of adult cases may be subclinical and not come to medical attention; the usual STD prevention measures such as using condoms, limiting the number of sexual partners, knowing one's sexual partners' infection status and partner notification will not be helpful. Often the sexual partner to be notified turns out to be the unrecognized source of infection.

For most of the same reasons, it is difficult to conceive of any effective control programme which is based upon timely identification of at risk individuals for pre- or post- exposure prophylaxis with vaccine and/or immune serum globulin. In addition, these individuals increasingly are socio-economically disadvantaged inner city minorities in whom sexual transmission of STD is at least partly driven by a vicious cycle of sex for drugs. Delivering routine preventive medicine of any kind to them has proven to be discouragingly problematic.

By a process of elimination, the only valid strategy to effectively control sexually transmitted hepatitis B in most countries is universal immunization of infants or young adolescents in school or both. This strategy is needed to provide immunity from infection before risk-taking behaviour is acquired and in persons with no known risk factors. Whether such an approach is cost/effective in a world of limited medical resources requires further analysis.

References

1. Alter MJ, Hadler SC, Margolis, et al (1990) JAMA 263: 1218.
2. Kane MI (1990) This volume.
3. Catterall RD (1978) Brit J Ven Dis 54: 335.
4. Schreeder MT, Thompson SE, Hadler SC, et al (1982) J Infect Dis 146: 7.
5. Reiner NE, Judson FN, Bond WW, et al (1982) Ann Intern Med 96: 170.

6. Francis DP, Hadler SC, Thompson SE, et al (1982) Ann Intern Med 97: 362.
7. Hadler SC, Judson FN, O'Malley PM, et al (1990) J Infect Dis (in press).
8. Judson FN (1981) Sex Transm Dis 8(S): 336.

Index of authors